MW00648918

DR. MARIOS MICHAEL, DC, CNS, cFMP

UNDERSTANDING
GENOMICS

How Nutrition, Supplements, and Lifestyle Can Help
You Unlock Your Genetic Superpowers

Print ISBN: 978-1-66782-400-0
eBook ISBN: 978-1-66782-401-7

Dedicated to my Wife, Elma, my love, and to our children Cool Lukas and Amazing Alice, for their unconditional love, support, and bountiful happiness. I am forever grateful.

TABLE OF CONTENTS

_____

A PEEK INSIDE PANDORA'S BOX

MY WIFE AND I FREQUENTLY EXERCISE TOGETHER, BUT WHETHER IT'S RUN-ning or riding bikes, she almost always outperforms me. She has the endurance of a champion. Even when it comes to keeping up with the kids, she always seems to have an advantage. We thought it was funny and could joke about it, but I'm also a competitive person, which motivated me to push myself harder. It wasn't until later when we found out why those activities always came easier to her than they did to me. It turned out that she actually did have an advantage that neither of us was aware of, and it was linked to her genes.

A couple of years ago, we both decided to try out 23andMe. Like the commercials advertise, you send in a swab of your DNA, and the results tell you about your heritage. It's a good conversation piece, and it's exciting to learn where you come from. I was born in Cyprus, so I thought I was 100 percent Cypriot, but it turns out that I'm 48 percent Sardinian. Who knew?

There is also a genetic component to the test. We learned many fun facts about eye color, taste buds, hair color, and a slew of other traits. What we found even more interesting was that it turned out that my wife had a common genetic mutation that allowed her to perform athletically.

The ACTN3 gene controls whether muscle cells produce a protein called alpha-actinin-3, found in fast-twitch muscle fibers. According to 23andMe, "While some people don't produce this protein at all, almost all of the elite power athletes who have been studied have a genetic variant that allows them to produce the protein. This suggests that the protein may be beneficial at least at the highest levels of power-based athletic competition."

I didn't have that gene, which on the surface seemed like a minor detail, but it made me realize that only a small difference in our genetic code could have such a significant impact on our bodies and how we function as humans. That got me thinking about what else I could learn by studying my genes.

I've always been curious about the human body—its functions, and how it can be improved naturally. That's why I became a chiropractor. Time and time again, I saw how making adjustments to the spine and removing obstructions could help the nervous system better send signals to and from the brain. Chiropractic school required taking a lot of nutrition courses. That further piqued my interest, and led me to expand my knowledge through seminars before becoming certified as a nutrition specialist. What followed was an interest in functional medicine. Now, for over 18 years, I've applied both nutrition and functional medicine to my practice and saw how much it helped my patients get better faster, stay healthier longer, and prevent certain conditions while managing their medication and its side effects.

Despite the great strides we've made in health care and nutrition, there is always room for improvement. I've watched people work so hard to reach retirement only to spend their time going from doctor to doctor and taking medication after medication, which prevented them from traveling and enjoying their kids and grandkids as they anticipated. That's why I continue to keep up on the latest scientific research, because I like to know what's coming and how I can use it to further help my patients. I have a personal drive to see how I can use science to set me apart from the other practitioners.

I learned about genomics when the Human Genome Project was completed in the early 2000s. For the first time ever, scientists were able to study the complete genetic blueprint of a human being. I was fascinated. Information was limited at first, but the field rapidly began to grow. I saw a shift taking place, and there was an opportunity with genomics that wasn't there before to truly personalize medicine. I set out to learn as much as possible, and completed a two-year certification in Genetics and Genomics at Stanford University, one of the leading universities in the field. I walked away from that course with the knowledge of how to use DNA, genetics, and nutrigenomics to further improve the level of care and treatment I could provide my patients. With functional medicine, I set out to treat the root cause of a particular disease, but with the inclusion of genomics, I would be able to take that one step further by identifying the pathway of those diseases to possibly prevent them from even developing.

It started small. The first patient I treated using genomics was an autistic boy who had traveled from overseas with his mother because they didn't have the resources where they were from. When I started to see results, my practice expanded. One female patient of mine went through three IVF procedures and couldn't get pregnant; each time, she suffered a miscarriage. She just wanted a child, and it wasn't happening, so her mother-in-law referred her to me. We did a genomic test and learned that she had several mutations, including a COMT mutation, which is a mutation that made her prone to miscarriages. I put her on a three-month detox and had her postpone her next IVF procedure until after the detox. We then created a food and supplement plan specific to her genes. The following IVF procedure was successful, and today she has a beautiful girl.

I've since gone on to treat hundreds of patients for conditions that include cardiovascular disease, high cholesterol, obesity, low testosterone, vitamin D deficiency, and cancer. I don't claim to have a cure for any of these diseases, but the paradigm has shifted in medicine: Your genes are no longer your destiny.

Did you know that if you have the GSTT1 gene mutation, there is an increased chance of getting certain cancers during your lifetime, because that gene keeps the cancer cells in your body low?[1] There is nothing we can do about that. Your genes don't change over time, but we can change how those genes are expressed—or turned on and off—through diet, supplementation, exercise, lifestyle, and outside environmental factors. If you know your genetic makeup and what conditions you might be predisposed to, you can use that information to give yourself a better chance of not developing those conditions. And if you do have certain conditions, knowing your genetic blueprint can change how you approach treatment.

I've tested the genome for some patients and discovered they had a mutation that impacted how they processed statin medication. They were then able to consult with their doctor to adjust their dosage and frequency to minimize side effects without altering the drug's effectiveness. That's the field of pharmacogenomics, and it's rapidly growing. The FDA has done extensive research on the genomic predisposition to certain medications and is starting to develop guidelines to determine the drugs and dosage for specific gene mutations.

Once you know your genetic information, you can improve your health immediately through simple changes. The main reason why people don't do it is that this information is not wildly available. It's also highly complex and difficult to understand, so they don't even try. That's where I hope to bridge the gap. I want to make this material simple and easy to understand, so you can begin making small changes to your daily life that will have a significant impact.

I'll bet you didn't know that you can immediately improve your health and well-being, starting today, merely by taking a different B-12 vitamin? The most common form of B-12 comes from a natural source called methylcobalamin, which can be found at almost any store that sells supplements. However, since 70 to 80 percent of the patients I've treated over the years have the MTHFR mutation, adenosyl/hydroxy B12 is more beneficial than the common B12 supplement. Not only is it natural, so it's absorbed and retained in the body differently, but it can help change the way specific gene mutations linked to widespread diseases are expressed. Just that one minor detail changes the science behind how you medicate yourself and can significantly impact your overall health, but so few people know about it.

Genomics can also be used to impact the world of sports and training. Doctors today can use genetics to determine an athlete's susceptibility to certain injuries, which allows them to train differently to prevent those injuries. Genetics is even responsible for an individual's own athletic ability. For example, those who have the same elite athlete gene as my wife should train differently than those who don't. They have fast-twitch muscle fibers compared to slow-twitch muscle fibers, which means they benefit from exercises (or a series of exercises) with quick bursts and fewer repetitions, such as circuit training and plyometrics. The more I work with clients, the more I've seen how adapting workouts according to their genetic makeup can improve their performance. What's funny is that now, whenever a new client walks into my office, I can usually tell if they possess that gene just by their stature, musculature, and the way they carry themselves.

Now that the cost of studying your DNA has significantly decreased and become affordable for the average person, genomics has become a significant part of what I do at my practice; but the medical world is only scratching the surface when it comes to learning what is possible. It's an exciting time in science and medicine because Pandora's Box is just starting to open, and we are getting our first peek inside, but there is no sugar coating it—genomics is complicated. I know because, even with a background in functional medicine and nutrition, I had many questions for my professors at Stanford. And the more I learned, the more questions I had.

Numerous studies have been done on a scientific level, but there has been very little written about the subject outside the scientific community, making this knowledge less accessible to the average person. We need to change that because everything derives from your genes—how you think, act, look, and feel. Your genes tell the story of who you are and how you function. They are a recipe for you. With that knowledge, you can take action now to enjoy longevity. You can learn what supplements and drugs are best for you and how much of them you should take to maximize effectiveness. That's important, because we're all different, and there is no one size that fits all solution. The more you know about your genes, the more you can personalize your health care. It's not far-fetched to believe that one day it will be common practice to have your genetic information on the front page of your file at the doctor's office. I believe that every aspect of medicine serves its purpose, and genomics is quickly becoming a part of the bigger picture. Genetics will not only help to make medicine more personalized, it will also make it more preventative because we won't just be treating the condition; we can work to prevent the condition from ever developing.

Over the past several hundred years, brilliant minds have collaborated and conducted experiments that helped us better understand and define genetics. That work continues, and great strides are being made every year. As technology advances, everything is getting more precise. Some of it sounds like science fiction. It won't be long before doctors can grow entire organs based on your genome, so your body won't reject them.[2] There is already a lot of work underway that studies the liver and kidneys. Scientists have created mutated pigs born with absolutely no kidneys and then injected the animal with the stem cells needed to grow fully functioning kidneys that their bodies don't reject because the organ is specific to the pig's personal genome.[3] In vitro fertilization allows us to insert the specific genes we want into a cell. It probably won't be long before it's scientifically possible to design a human being, but that power raises a whole host of ethical concerns and questions. It's startling to think where this technology is headed, but simultaneously it's so exciting to see that we're pushing the boundaries of what we once thought was possible.

That's where this book comes in. The subject matter may be complicated, but this book is written for the average person—the one without a science background. Research is cited, but I've taken the overly technical and scientific explanations out of the text, so you don't need to be an expert to understand it. There is much more to the complex world of genomics than what is contained in these pages, but my goal is for you to walk away with a clear understanding of this new field. I will answer all of the questions that my clients ask me, and I've been asked a lot of questions over the years. What are genes? What is DNA? What is genomics? How can I make my genes work for me? If I take one of these tests, is my DNA raw data protected? If I have certain diseases running in my family, how do I protect myself?

I'm going to explain how what you put in your body and outside environmental factors can affect your genes. This book will bridge the gap between science, genomics, nutrition, and supplementation, so you can learn how to make your genes work for you. Think of this as both a resource and a step-by-step guide that provides all the options at your disposal to help you unlock the power of your genes and live a healthier life. Everything I recommend is something that I've personally seen work. I don't have an affiliation with any of the companies or organizations mentioned. When I talk about supplements, they are the supplements I've taken, my family has taken, and my patients have taken. It's worked for us, and it can work for you!

PART I

THE SCIENCE: BOILED DOWN AND SIMPLIFIED

CHAPTER 1:

DNA: THE HUMAN BLUEPRINT

You've all heard of DNA, and you've seen the double helix, but do you really know what DNA is and what it does? Yes, DNA is the blueprint for a living organism, be it a human being or a houseplant. It's the basis for our existence, and just like a good recipe book, it contains all of the instructions for creating the proteins in our bodies. In essence, it contains what makes you uniquely you. But what is it? How does it work?

DNA, or deoxyribonucleic acid, is a molecule. Think of it like a six-billion-letter code that provides the assembly instructions for everything from eye color to why you might be susceptible to cancer. All of that can be found in your DNA.

Nucleotides are what make up DNA, and they have three main parts:

- Sugar
- Phosphate
- Nucleic acid or base pairs
  - ▷ These base pairs are made up of four key amino acids:
    - · Adenine (A)
    - · Thymine (T)

· Cytosine (C)

· Guanine (G)

  ▪ These bases are paired in the middle and held together by hydrogen bonds.

    • A pairs with T

    • C pairs with G

These nucleotides are structured in two long strands that create a spiral called the double helix. A double-helix structure resembles a ladder, with the nucleotide base pairs forming the ladder's rungs while the sugar and phosphate molecules create the ladder's vertical sidepieces, or the backbone.

The National Institutes of Health (NIH) came up with an analogy that I like and that might help you think of how this works. There are 26 letters in the English alphabet—A through Z—but the alphabet for our genes has only four letters—A, C, G, and T. Just like the letters of the English language come together to tell a story, so do the letters of our genes.

Our DNA comprises about 6.4 billion letters (or 3.2 billion bases) long, and approximately 99.9 percent of those bases are similar in all people. Each DNA strand is almost six feet (1.8 meters long) but is crammed into a space of just 0.09 micrometers.[4]

FUN FACT:

One gram of DNA has the capability of storing 700 terabytes of data. That's almost equal to 14,000 Blu-ray disks.[5]

GENES, RNA, & PROTEINS

A gene is a stretch of DNA that is a code for a trait or an organism's specific characteristic. These genetic traits can determine if you have seemingly innocuous features like blue eyes, freckles, dimples, or much more serious traits, such as a predisposition to certain conditions and diseases. A single strand of DNA contains thousands of genes, and humans have roughly 20,000 to 25,000 genes of all sizes.[6]

The gene is first expressed into RNA (ribonucleic acid). RNA is a recipe for building protein and a partial copy of the DNA code. It's similar to DNA, but it's a smaller, single strand that is only one side of the DNA ladder yet still contains identical base pairs of that DNA strand. RNA has sugar ribose instead of deoxyribose, and instead of a thymine base, RNA uses uracil.

These RNA strands fit into a RIBOSOME, and it's the ribosome's job to read the RNA code, gather amino acids (there are over 20 different types of amino acids of all different shapes), and stick them together as part of a code to form a protein.

In the genetics world, the central dogma is that the DNA makes the RNA, and the RNA makes the proteins. There are millions of different proteins, and they use the instructions provided by the gene to do the work of expressing a particular trait.

FUN FACT:

A gene is usually 10,000 nucleotides long. It encodes the protein, which may have up to 3,000 nucleotides in its RNA.

Those proteins are a guide that gives our cells, tissues, organs, and organ systems much of their structure and function. Proteins do thousands of jobs (including breaking down food, building and replacing tissue, and cell division) that influence how our body works and shape our individual characteristics.

In other words, genes provide the instruction manual to create YOU, both the good and the not so good. These unique recipes are transferred from parents to children, which explains the occurrence of certain inherited diseases. Think of it like this:

- Amino acids form proteins.
- Proteins form living cells.
- Living cells form tissues.
- Tissues form organs.

Functionally related organs often work together to form organ systems. There are 11 integrated major organ systems in the human organism:

1. Integumentary/Exocrine
2. Skeletal
3. Muscular
4. Nervous
5. Endocrine
6. Circulatory/Cardiovascular
7. Immune/Lymphatic
8. Respiratory
9. Digestive
10. Urinary
11. Reproductive

FUN FACT:

Different creatures have different genes, but the basic DNA code is similar for all living things. For example, humans and chimps share 99 percent of their DNA.[7]

CHROMOSOMES

When DNA is compacted and wrapped around protein structures, it can be organized into a chromosome. Almost all of our DNA is arranged into chromosomes, and there are roughly between 500 and 4,000 genes per chromosome. Humans have 46 chromosomes in each cell of the body—23 pairs—with half inherited from the mother and half inherited from the father.

Chromosomes are made from chromatin, which is the packaging DNA comes in. Chromatin is comprised of DNA and clusters of proteins called HISTONES.

These histones give the protein structure and also help to regulate gene expression. We have 30 million of these molecule spools in each of our cells.[8] DNA coiled around eight histones form nucleosomes. This helps package the DNA, but it also prevents some of the genes from being accessible. The cell can't always read them, so not all genes are active all the time. Depending on if this coil loosens or tightens, genes can be turned on and off—something we will get into more detail about later. Just know for now that even though we may not be able to change or control our genes, we can control the gene expression.

FUN FACT:

The word "chromosome" is derived from the Greek words "Khroma" and "soma," which mean color and body.

CELLS

Everything we've discussed is contained within the cell. Proteins come together to form living cells, each with 46 strands of DNA. Our body has approximately 10 to 100 trillion cells, each with different functions. And each cell has roughly six feet of DNA.[9] The cell nuclei contain 99.9 percent of our genes, and roughly 0.1 percent are within the mitochondria.[10]

Not all genes are active all the time, and it's the cell's job to control which genes are turned on and off. Different types of cells need different genes expressed. Skin cells provide a protective barrier and produce skin color. Nerve cells transfer messages. Digestive cells help with digestion. And so forth.

The instructions in your DNA are translated into a language known as the genetic code. The cells divide the bases into triplets known as codons, which are code words for amino acids that tell the cells what to make and when to start and stop reading.[11]

GENOME

Together, the DNA, genes, and chromosomes make up the genome, or the complete set of genes in an organism.

The genome contains all the instructions and information needed for an organism to form, maintain itself, and function. We have a copy of that genome in every cell of our body. Every human has a unique genome containing genes that determine things like height, eye color, and whether you may be susceptible to certain diseases. Our genomes are 99.9 percent identical to every other human being on the planet, but it's that 0.1 percent that amounts to 3.1 million different ways that we can be different from each other genetically.[12]

The vast majority of our DNA still remains a mystery to scientists. In fact, 98.5 percent of DNA sequences are what's called "junk DNA," which for a long period of time scientists thought was useless.[13] The term was coined by the late geneticist Susumu Ohno in 1972, but is falling out of favor now because discoveries show that this "junk DNA" can evolve into functional DNA. The late Stephen Jay Gould and paleontologist Elisabeth Vrba at Yale University have since revealed how junk DNA may take on a new role.[14] They can make these discoveries simply because they have access to more information as we learn more about this fascinating arena.

FUN FACT:
One genome is equal to one terabyte (1 TB) that would allow you to download 286,000 iTunes songs, 416,000 photos (300 dpi), and a Word document containing 16,500,000 words.[15]

GENOMICS

GENETICS is the study of the role genes play in inheritance and how certain traits and conditions are passed down from one generation to another.

GENOMICS means "all of the genes," and is the study of those letters in our DNA (A, C, G, and T) and how each string of letters passes information to help each cell in your body work properly.

While genetics focuses on individual genes, genomics focuses on all of the genes together—their interaction together and with the organism's environment. Genomics includes the scientific study of complex diseases—such as heart disease, asthma, diabetes, and cancer—as these diseases are typically caused more by a combination of genetic and environmental factors than by individual genes. Genomics offers new possibilities for therapies and treatments for some complex diseases as well as new diagnostic methods.

I like to think of genomics as prevention at its best. There is a history of cardiovascular disease on my father's side of my family, and when I tested my DNA, I learned that sure enough, I inherited specific genes linked to heart disease and cardiovascular disease. I was in my forties at the time and had no symptoms, but knowing that I was predisposed to those conditions allowed me to take the necessary precautions.

Outside environmental factors can influence whether certain genes are expressed (such as epigenetics, which we'll discuss later). But through nutrition, supplementation, and lifestyle, we can give your body a better chance to prevent certain genetic mutations that might predispose us to certain conditions.

FUN FACT:
If a person worked eight hours a day typing 60 words-per-minute, it would take them almost 50 years to type the entire human genome.[16]

THE HUMAN GENOME PROJECT

So much of the information we know today is a result of the Human Genome Project.

In 1990, the Human Genome Project was initiated by the U.S. Department of Energy and the National Institutes of Health (NIH), and involved countries all over the world, including England, China, and Germany. They laid out what became known as the Bermuda Principles to ensure that all of the countries involved worked together and shared data. Thirteen years and $3 billion later, the project accomplished its mission to map all of the DNA in a human cell.[17]

David Haussler and Jim Kent built the first-ever web-based tool for reading and sharing the genome online for anyone to study. The project identified each of the human genes, but we are still learning what they all mean. This became a massive source of information for researchers in the fields of science and medicine. As Director of the U.S. National Human Genome Research Institute, Dr. Francis Collins, MD, Ph.D., said, "Sequencing the human genome is not an end in itself, it is just the start of a revolution in genomics and genetics that will change the face of medicine in the twenty-first century."[18]

A lot has changed since 1990, and with advanced technology, the process is much faster today.

FUN FACT:

If you somehow managed to unwind all of the DNA molecules from a single human body and place them end-to-end, they would span a whopping length of 10 billion miles, which is almost the same distance between the Earth and Pluto.[19]

GENE MUTATIONS

We all start our lives as mutants!

This isn't always a bad thing. In fact, it's very common. A mutation is a change that occurs in our DNA sequence, either because of a mistake when the DNA is copied or because of environmental factors. This is where the (±) comes in. If a gene is normal and there is no mutation, that's designated with a (−). If a mutation is present, that is designated with a (+). Remember, we inherit two copies of every gene—one from each parent—so you might get a (+) from one parent and a (−) from the other.

- Homozygous (+/+): You've inherited two mutated genes, one from each parent.
- Homozygous (−/−): You've inherited two normal genes, one from each parent.
- Heterozygous (+/−): You've inherited a mutated gene from one parent and a normal gene from another.

Mutations can be broken down into two main categories:

1. NULL MUTATIONS

Remember that a gene is a prescription to make RNA, and the RNA carries the instructions to make the protein. Genes are 10,000 nucleotides long. They encode the protein, which may have 3,000 nucleotides in its RNA. What null mutations (or deletion mutations) do is basically kill the entire gene, so there is no protein being made. In this case, there is nothing you can do.

2. OTHER MUTATIONS (Non-Null Mutations)

These other mutations only affect a portion of those 10,000 nucleotides, and the outcome depends entirely on which and how many of those nucleotides are affected.

This is also where chromatin comes into play, because how tight that histone coil is wrapped around the proteins will determine how much of that gene is expressed. So, if the mutation causes the gene to be down 40 percent, a tight coil could cause it to be down 60 percent or more. However, the opposite is true as well. If the chromatin is loose and opens up, it might offset that 40 percent, so even though you have a mutation, it compensates for the loss and becomes a normal functioning gene. In other words, the state of chromatin can control the gene expression by being too tight or too loose. The basis for this is epigenetics, which we will go into in much more detail in the next chapter.

There are three examples of non-null mutations.

1. Partial: This is a mutation that weakens, but doesn't eliminate, the gene, so it can end up with 10 percent activity rather than 0 percent. These are often referred to as "W" for weak.

2. Increased: This is a mutation that increases the activity of the gene, such as a mutation in a growth receptor that causes the gene to always be active and the cells to grow. This type of mutation is often involved in cancer, such as the HER2 growth factor receptor, which causes breast cancer.

3. Altered: This mutation gives the gene a new function, such as in the gene for Huntington's disease. The Huntington mutation is a triplet DNA repeat that forces the Huntington protein to have many more Q amino acids. This causes the proteins to glom together and form protein tangles in your

neurons. This eventually kills the neurons and causes the disease, which prevents you from moving your muscles.

Diving deeper into various subcategories of mutations, there are also:

*GERMLINE MUTATIONS: These are inheritable mutations that you can pass along to your offspring. They occur during the chromosomal arrangement. Traits like blue eyes, red hair, and a "unibrow" are germline mutations. Some diseases like Down syndrome and autism fit into this category as well. These mutations cannot be changed. You might be able to help the condition to a certain extent, but you can't reverse it—at least not yet.

*SOMATIC MUTATIONS: These are the types of mutations, like certain forms of cancer and other diseases, that are impacted by epigenetics, and occur in the cells of your body. They are not passed down to the next generation. However, many inherited diseases are rare because they are typically recessive, which means they need to have two copies of the mutated gene (+/+), one from each parent, to inherit the disease.

Most of our gene mutations were discovered during the completion of the Human Genome Project. Researchers learned that people with a particular type of mutation tended to develop certain diseases or traits more often. Gene mutations can have varying effects on health depending on where they occur and if they change the function of the proteins. The most common types of mutations are:

1. POINT MUTATIONS: This is where one DNA base letter changes to another. It's a change of only one letter, which may not seem like a lot, but try thinking of it how it was explained to me at Stanford. What if I gave you the following instructions: "Get one cup of 'milk,' add two teaspoons of chocolate, stir until mixed thoroughly. Now change the "m" in milk to an "s."[20] Adding one cup of silk to two teaspoons of chocolate gives you a completely different result. Sickle cell anemia is a serious disease that results from only a single change to one letter in the genetic code.

2.   INSERTIONS OR DELETIONS: Small bits of DNA are added or missing, as in Huntington's disease. Piggybacking on that same example above, imagine those same instructions if the word "milk" was deleted altogether. That would lead to a completely different issue and outcome. The same thing happens with insertions. It would be like the phrase "get one cup of milk" was repeated. Cystic fibrosis is an example, which is caused by a single deletion.

3.   REARRANGEMENTS: This is when the chromosomes are completely rearranged, so if you changed the words in the sentence above to "milk one get of cup," it wouldn't mean anything. Charcot-Marie Tooth disease Type 1 is an example of this type of mutation.

FUN FACT:

In the scientific community, there is a difference between a "mutation" and a "variation." Many use them interchangeably, but the difference is: "The changes in the nucleotide sequence at the DNA level or in any one of the base pairs is known as a mutation, while the genetic variation is how one individual of a species variate from another. Variation can be due to changes in the nucleotide sequence like insertions, deletions, and genetic rearrangements or any environmental factors."[21]

SNPs

The most common and most studied genetic mutations are SNPs, or single nuclear polymorphisms.

They are so common that SNPs occur almost once in every 1,000 nucleotides, translating to four to five million SNPs in a person's genome. And as mentioned, these mutations can be benign features or crippling diseases. Having a gene with an SNP mutation doesn't mean that the gene is nonfunctioning or defective. It just means that it's functioning with a different efficiency—sometimes at a lower level, sometimes at a higher level, and sometimes it lacks regulatory mechanisms commonly involved at its expression.

A genetic mutation may impact how much of a particular cell's protein is expressed, thus altering that cell's function and the system it's part of. Remember, cells make tissue, tissue makes organs, and organs make systems. A mutation also impacts the switches that control when and where a protein is active and how much of it is made. For example, lactase is an enzyme that helps infants break down lactose, or the sugar in milk. Normally, the gene that codes for lactase is turned off around age four, so when those who don't make lactase consume milk, they experience gastrointestinal issues. Those with a mutation that keeps the lactase gene active (lactase persistence), can digest milk as adults.[22] Recently, another gene has been identified, which tells us if someone is likely to develop lactose intolerance later in life as an adult.

A GLIMPSE INTO THE FUTURE

There have been some incredible advances in DNA sequencing, and the CRISPR/Cas9 method is one of the most significant because it uses bacteria that can actually edit the DNA of every species, even humans.

Clustered Regularly Interspaced Short Palindromic Repeats, or CRISPR/Cas9, was first introduced by Emmanuelle Charpentier and Jennifer Doudna in 2012, and is now considered one of the most important discoveries in the history of biology. This is targeted genome editing that allows you to actually snip genes. It can find where the bad gene is, cut it out, and reconnect it. Genomics today is getting that precise. The process involves programming bacteria that literally go into the arm of a chromosome, cut it, remove the mutation, and permanently attach the other end of the DNA so the organism can go on living without the mutation. The process continues to be fine-tuned and refined. More recent discoveries show that nanobodies (single-domain antibodies) can be used to help CRISPR turn certain genes on and off.[23]

This technology is a significant improvement over the former genome-editing tools and reaches completely new heights of targeting, effectiveness, and ease of use. Previous methods weren't accurate and could create additional mutations when trying to cut other genes. The CRISPR/Cas9 method is 99 percent accurate and permanent.

There are some ethical questions, but the potential for this as a therapeutic is enormous because it could remove mutations that can lead to certain diseases. Technology moves so fast that there is a good chance that it won't be long before even the information prevented here is improved upon.

CHAPTER 2:

EPIGENETICS—HOW GENES CAN BE TURNED ON AND OFF

WHEN PEOPLE SAY THAT YOUR GENES AREN'T YOUR DESTINY, THEY ARE talking about epigenetics, which is the study of gene expression that does not involve alterations to the DNA sequence. The word derives from the Greek word "epi," which means above—so it's above your DNA.

There are three prevalent views of what epigenetics truly is: chromatin changes, methylation (which we'll dive into in the next section), and outside environmental factors. No matter how you define epigenetics, if your DNA sequence is nature, epigenetics is nurture. It's how your diet, lifestyle, and outside environmental factors can determine whether or not that gene mutation is expressed, meaning whether a particular gene is turned on or off.

If you have a (−/−), that means you've inherited two healthy genes, and there is no mutation present. If you have a (+/−), that means the gene could go in either direction. Even if you have a (+/+), and there is a mutation present, epigenetics can limit, if not downright silence, the expression of that gene.

The other side of the coin is true as well, and you can just as easily make it worse with your behavior and the outside factors you are exposed to. This means that you are in more control of your genes than you might think. How is any of this possible?

Let's do a deeper dive and go back to the very beginning—the creation of the cell. All of the cells in our bodies started from a single cell sharing the same DNA, which after many divisions, left us with over 200 different cell types and 50 to 100 trillion cells.[24]

The more you think about this, the more questions you might have. Like, if all the cells in our bodies started from a single cell sharing the exact DNA, then why don't all of our cells look and behave the same? For instance, why do our heart cells look different than our ear cells? Why would one identical twin have a disease when the other twin with the exact same DNA does not? How can there be one genome but a different expression of genes?

The reason is that it's not just our genes that determine who we are. It's our environment. This is where epigenetics comes in, which is the study of how DNA interacts with the smaller group of molecules within cells to activate and deactivate certain genes. To access the DNA information within individual cells and create proteins, a gene must be "expressed," which means that it must either be turned ON or OFF.

Most proteins remain in the cell, but once a gene is expressed, under normal circumstances, the protein is transferred out of our cells and starts specific tasks based on the information provided by the particular gene. In the case of heart cells and ear cells, different proteins were turned on or off, which gave us the different organs and specific organ functions—ears primarily for hearing and heart primarily for pumping blood throughout our body.

When trying to understand epigenetics, a useful analogy is to compare genes with a recipe book, since genes are like recipes for specific tasks. In a recipe book, all of the information can be used to make different dishes. However, we only use the apple pie recipe for apple pie. Similarly, we only use those genes needed in an ear to make an ear, even though our DNA contains thousands of recipes. In essence, the epigenetic process tells the cells to read specific pages of the instruction manual at specific times. Epigenetics is a relatively new study in genetics, but it is very empowering, and it puts us in the driver seat of our genetic destiny.

Another analogy is to picture how a symphony performance comes together. If the DNA is the sheet music, any alterations during the conductor's performance or the musicians are like the epigenetic changes, and the end result, or the performance that the audience watches, is like the human trait. Those traits are phenotypes, such as blue eyes, height, or even a susceptibility to certain diseases. All phenotypes result from a combination of multiple genes.

Assistant Professor of Pediatrics at Boston Children's Hospital, and recent recipient of the Presidential Early Career Award for Scientists and Engineers (PECASE), Dr. Eric Greer, MD, said, "Epigenetics is what enables every cell to act differently, despite having the same DNA, based on their needs and in response to the environment."[25] It's this process that is regulated by epigenetics, and it's what I like to call *THE DIFFERENCE MAKER.*

EPIGENETIC CHANGES

Different from a mutation, which is a permanent change to your DNA, your genes can also undergo reversible changes, and those are called epigenetic changes—whether it be a chromatin state modification (open or closed), environmental change, the gray area of methylation, or a hybrid where environmental changes affect the chromatin state via methylation. These changes are actually a common and natural occurrence that can be influenced by several environmental factors, such as:

- Stress
- Age
- Lifestyle
- Food
- Bacteria
- Gut health
- Lack of sleep

- Lack of touch
- Lack of exercise
- Fear
- Alcohol
- High-fat diet
- Sugar

FUN FACT:

One suspected environmental trigger to affect the behavior of an organism's epigenome is a chemical found in many plastic bottles, include baby bottles, called bisphenol-A.

Some epigenetic changes can be a result of DNA damage (nature) from outside environmental or nutritional factors and conditions a person is exposed to, called exposomes. Some examples are:

- Toxins
- Free radicals
- Ultraviolet radiation
- Chemicals
- Viruses
- Infections

"Exposome" is a word being mentioned a lot lately, and with good reason, because it's not just your genes that are important; it's how your genes interact with your environment that really matters. That's why people are right when they say that health is a state between your genome and your exposome.

Mutations can also be caused by reactive oxygen species (ROS), which are the byproducts of food and environmental toxins that can wreak havoc on our genes and DNA. ROS occurs when inflammation is present and over-powers antioxidant nutrients in the body. ROS is an imbalance in antioxidant production and pro-oxidant production, which can react with proteins and lead to tissue damage and genomic instability in the form of mutations and altered cellular function. [26]

The way this works goes back to the DNA that's wrapped around histone proteins in the cell. Depending on how tight the strand of DNA wraps around each histone, it can turn sets of genes on or off. If wrapped tight, it protects the DNA information, so it can remain dormant. If loose, that information is more vulnerable. This causes various epigenetic changes, and it is linked to everything including the food we eat, exercise, and environmental factors. This is how you can amplify either the (+) or the (−) of a particular gene. Knowing that puts you more in control over which genes are expressed.

Today, we know of five types of epigenetic changes (all nurture):

1. Methylation—Methyl groups are added to the DNA molecule.

2. Acetylation—The addition of an acetyl group.

3. Phosphorylation—The attachment of a phosphoryl group.

4. Ubiquitylation—Protein inactivation by adding ubiquitin to it, aka the "kiss of death" process for a protein.

5. Sumoylation—This plays an essential functional role in the DNA damage response.

METHYLATION

Methylation gets the most attention, and rightfully so because it's the most frequent and the most important. Out of all of the epigenetic changes, it's the one we know the most about—by far!

About 96 percent of the mass of the human body is made up of oxygen, carbon, hydrogen, and nitrogen (with most of that being water). The rest involves carbon atoms bound to carbon, hydrogen, nitrogen, and oxygen. A methyl group is a single carbon atom bound only to hydrogen, and methylation (or one-carbon metabolism) is the transfer of these methyl groups.[27]

Methylation is a vital metabolic biochemical process that occurs in every cell of our bodies when a chemical unit called a methyl group (which contains one carbon and three hydrogen atoms) is added to cytosine—one of the four bases of a DNA molecule. This happens a billion times a second.[28] Methyl groups transfer from one molecule to another (as one group releases the molecule and the other absorbs it), which can then activate or deactivate certain substances like an on/off switch. Methylation is essential for life, and we need it for survival. It contributes to detoxification, energy production, inflammation control, mood balancing, hormone metabolization, DNA repair, and glutathione production, and has been linked to longevity. It also helps to produce:

- Serotonin
- Melatonin
- Glutathione
- Nitric oxide
- Coenzyme Q10
- Epinephrine
- Cysteine
- Norepinephrine
- Taurine
- L-carnitine[29]

Methylation was first believed to shut down dangerous stretches of DNA that could move from their original position on the chromosomes to other parts of the genome in ways that caused disease. We've since learned that methylation also helps regulate the activity of normal genes, and that it can go awry in many cancers and other diseases.

FUN FACT:

A methyl group is one of the simplest atomic arrangements in organic chemistry, because it consists of only one carbon atom and three hydrogen atoms.

ARE YOU OVER-OR UNDER-METHYLATED?

The MTHFR gene provides instructions for making an enzyme called methylenetetrahydrofolate reductase. This plays a role in processing amino acids, which are the building blocks of proteins. Methylenetetrahydrofolate reductase is important for a chemical reaction involving the vitamin folate, also called vitamin B9. The key nutrients in the methylation system include:

- Methionine
- Homocysteine
- Vitamin A
- Vitamin B1, B2, B3, B6, B9, B12
- Choline
- Betaine (TMG)
- Glycine
- Minerals: Iron, Phosphorus, Sulfur, Magnesium, Potassium, Zinc, Cobalt

In my experience, approximately 60 to 80 percent of patients I have tested have an MTHFR or related mutation (+/−) or (+/+) that can lead to methylation disorder. This can accelerate aging, raise the risk of disease, and lead to numerous health issues, such as:

- Abnormal immune functionAllergies
- Alzheimer's disease
- Anemia
- Anxiety
- Arthritis
- Asthma
- Autism
- Autoimmune disease
- Behavior and learning disorders
- Cancer
- Cardiovascular disease
- Chronic fatigue
- Chronic infection

- Chronic inflammation
- Dementia
- Depression
- Diabetes
- Down syndrome
- Elevated blood pressureElevated blood sugarFood and chemical sensitivities
- Infertility, pregnancy problems, and miscarriage
- Insomnia
- Multiple sclerosis
- Neurotransmitter imbalance
- Obsessive-compulsive disorder
- Psychiatric disorders
- Racing thoughts
- Weight gain

These are the genes most commonly associated with the methylation pathway, and these are the diseases linked to these genes when they aren't functioning properly:

- SHMT: Infection, cell disrepair, wrinkles, inflamed gut, lack of new brain cells, and stress.
- MTR/MTRR: Neutral tube defects, disabilities conceiving, lack of B12, lack of energy, cancer, pernicious anemia, and not waking from anesthesia.
- BHMT: Decreased energy.
- AHCY: Decreased muscle tone.
- CBS: Higher levels of ammonia, which can lead to tremors, disorientation, brain fog, hyperactive reflexes, activation of NMDA receptors leading to glutamate excitotoxicity, paranoia, panic attacks, memory loss, hyperventilation, CNS toxicity, and Alzheimer's disease.
- SUOX: Higher levels of sulfites, sensitivity to sulfites, acid reflux, and migraines.

- MTHFR: Heart disease, neutral tube defects, disabilities conceiving, and cancer.

The methylation pathway is also linked to the following:

- Increased homocysteine: Renal failure, stroke, heart attack, diabetes, Alzheimer's disease, and natural defects.
- Decreased methylation: Cancer, aging, cardiovascular disease, neurological issues, retroviral transmission, neural defects, and Down syndrome.
- Decreased BH4: Diabetes, atypical phenylketonuria, decreased dopamine levels, decreased serotonin levels, hypertension, atherosclerosis, decreased NOS, and endothelial dysfunction.[30]
- Decreased estrogen detoxification: Increased susceptibility to postmenopausal estrogen sensitive cancers and overall prostate cancer risk.[31]
- Increased mitochondrial dysfunction: Aging, autism, bipolar disorder, schizophrenia, depression, diabetes, Parkinson's disease, asthma, chronic fatigue syndrome, Alzheimer's disease, gastrointestinal disorders, and a lack of energy.[32]

Proper methylation is dependent on various nutrients, and depending on which nutrients are deficient will determine if you are under- or over-methylated. Although statistics may vary, it is believed that 70 percent of the population exhibits normal methylation, while 22 percent are under-methylated and 8 percent are over methylated. It's believed that roughly 70 percent of those with mental disorders are either over- or under-methylated.[33] Certain conditions and symptoms are linked to being both under- and over-methylated, so you want to be right in the middle.

Some of the characteristics and traits of under-methylation include but are not limited to:

- OCD tendencies, ritualistic behavior.
- Addictiveness.
- Perfectionism.

- Self-motivated, strong-willed, and accomplished.
- Competitive.
- Calm demeanor, but inner tension and gloomy.
- Not showing emotions.
- Lack of empathy.
- Poor concentration.
- Antisocial.
- Oily skin and high fluidity.
- Strong teeth.
- Low homocysteine.
- Phobias.
- Denial and prone to delusions or conspiratorial theories.
- Slenderness.
- Seasonal allergies, but few food allergies.
- Low tolerance for pain.
- Frequent headaches and muscle cramps.
- Weak hair growth.
- High body temperature.
- Responds well to antihistamines and SSRIs.
- Low tolerance for alcohol.
- Low serotonin and dopamine.
- High libido.

Under-methylation is associated with the following issues:[34]

- 98% of those on the Autism Spectrum are under-methylated.
- 95% of those with Antisocial Personality Disorder are under-methylated.
- 90% of those with Schizoaffective Disorder are under-methylated
- 85% of those with Oppositional–Defiance are under-methylated.
- 82% of those with Anorexia are under-methylated.
- 38% of those with Depression are under-methylated.

Some of the characteristics and traits of over-methylation include, but are not limited to:

- Low motivation in school.
- Artistic or musical.
- Non-competitive.
- High anxiety or nervousness.
- High self-esteem.
- Hyperactive.
- Prone to self-mutilation.
- Believe that people think ill of them.
- Cheerful and grandiose.
- Prone to sleep disorders.
- Extrovert. Enjoys attention.
- Overly empathetic.
- Prone to hyperactivity.
- Obsessions without compulsions.
- Low libido.
- Good short-term memory.
- Tendency to be overweight.
- High tolerance to pain.
- History of eczema and dry skin.
- Absence of seasonal allergies, but several food and chemical allergies.
- Low histamine and antihistamine intolerance.
- Adverse reaction to SSRIs.
- Strong hair growth.
- Upper body, head, and neck pain.
- Elevated serotonin/dopamine activity.
- Food and chemical sensitivities.

Over-methylation is associated with the following issues:[35]

- 98 percent of those with panic or anxiety disorder are over-methylated.
- 52 percent of those with paranoid schizophrenia are over-methylated.

- 28 percent of those with ADHD are over-methylated.
- 30 percent of those with behavior disorders are over-methylated.
- 18 percent of those with depression (adverse reaction to SSRI medication) are over-methylated.

So, how can you find out where you stand?

Methylation can be measured, and there is a test to determine if you are under- or over-methylated. You could do a CHIP sequence, which is similar to a genomic analysis, but that's expensive. Keep in mind that any of these tests have to be prescribed by a medical professional. You can't do it on your own, but these are some of the potential options.

CONVENTIONAL LABS

- Next Enzymatic Methyl-seq Kit
- EpigenDx
- Qiagen—QIAseq Targeted Methyl Panels

FUNCTIONAL MEDICINE LABS

- Genova Diagnostics: Methylation Panel
- Doctor's Data: Methylation Panel

What I like about the functional medicine labs is that they offer two separate reports—one for the doctor and another that simplifies the findings for the patient. And there is a lot of explanation. Since interest continues to grow around this new science, the more conventional labs are beginning to provide the same detailed explanation for patients to help them better understand the complex data.

THE BUMBLEBEE EXPERIMENT

One of the most fascinating examples of environmentally controlled gene expression is an experiment done on bumblebees.[36] All bumblebee larvae have an identical DNA sequence, but one bee can be raised to be a worker and another to be a queen. How does that work? The answer lies in methylation.

The bee destined to become the queen is fed large amounts of royal jelly, which helps it develop unique communication skills, the instinct to kill rival queens, and a larger abdomen and ovaries for laying eggs. The worker bees are fed much less of the royal jelly and have rudimentary ovaries that practically render them sterile.

Scientists determined that once the baby bees are fed large amounts of royal jelly, it actually silences a key gene called Dnmt3 DNA Methyltransferase, so those baby bees develop into queens. When Dnmt3 is turned on, the opposite occurs, and the baby bees develop into workers.

It has been scientifically shown that the process is mediated by an epigenetic mark modification of DNA known as CpG methylation. The majority of bees with reduced DNA methylation levels emerged with the queen's characteristics. This finding suggests that epigenetics, through DNA methylation in bumblebees, allows for different expressions with the help of food.

FUN FACT:

Humans share somewhere between 40 and 50 percent of their DNA with cabbages. A recessive trait is passed down for generations, but visibly shows up after skipping several generations.[37]

THE AGOUTI GENE

As mammals, we all have the agouti gene. It's a hair color gene that may also affect appetite and activity. Scientists performed experiments in genetically identical twin mice (with identical genes), which showed us how important a mother's diet is in shaping her offspring's epigenome.[38]

When a mother's diet is rich in dietary methyl from food—such as asparagus, avocado, broccoli, Brussels sprouts, green leafy vegetables, legumes (peas, beans, lentils)—a mouse's agouti gene is methylated (as it is in normal mice), which helps to produce a brown coat of fur and a low risk for disease, diabetes, and obesity.

The same is not true for the mice with an unmethylated agouti gene. Those mice are more likely to develop a yellow coat of fur, become morbidly obese, and succumb to diabetes and cancer. Both mice—the yellow, fat, disease-prone, and the skinny, brown, healthy mice—are genetically identical with the same DNA. Their genome is exactly the same, but the gene expression is obviously different because of methylation.

The fat, yellow, disease-prone mice had an epigenetic mutation expressed by what the mother ate. The normal, healthy mice's agouti genes were kept in the "off" position by the epigenome (environment, diet), which allowed attachment of methyl groups to the corresponding regions of DNA (methylation). In the yellow, obese, disease-prone mice, the same genes were expressed or turned "on," which resulted in the unmethylated regions of DNA. The mice whose agouti gene was turned on are also more likely to suffer from diabetes and cancer as adults. This is an example of how what a mother eats can impact her offspring and, subsequently, even their health as an adult.

A different Stanford University study[39] on rats determined that you can pass not only your genes onto your offspring and future generations, but also certain behavioral changes, such as fear. Since we can't go back in time and change what our parents ate decades earlier, we can and should change what we eat now for optimum gene health. Maybe it's time to update the saying, "you are what you eat" to "you are what your parents and grandparents ate."

This is no longer speculation. Studies have concluded that, not only were the offspring born to mothers who were pregnant during the Dutch famine of 1944 smaller in statue, but so were the grandchildren of those offspring, even though their parents had a normal diet. Similar studies looked at the population of a small Swedish town during periods of both feast and famine. They found similar results, which show that the health of the mother during pregnancy has an impact on future generations.[40] Our genes take direction from our behaviors and habits.

The good news is that many of these typical changes aren't permanent and are reversible when methyl is back within normal range.[41] With the advancements in medicine and molecular biology, the idea that our genes are set in stone has been refuted. In fact, scientists have discovered that through epigenetics, we can determine how genes are turned on and off and what traits/variations to express, or even whether to be expressed at all, therefore controlling our genetic destiny.

FUN FACT:

The human agouti gene, which is 85 percent identical to the mouse's agouti gene, is expressed much more widely, including in adipose tissue (fat), testis, ovary, and heart, and at lower levels in the liver, kidney, and foreskin.[42]

PART II

THE PROCESS OF UNLOCKING YOUR GENES

CHAPTER 3:

GENOTYPING: READING OUR DNA

THE FIRST STEP TO UNLOCKING THE POWER OF YOUR GENES IS TO ACQUIRE your DNA raw data. This is easier today than ever before since technology has advanced to the point where that data is readily available, and the process is affordable. The cost of sequencing an entire human genome was around $100,000,000 in 2001, but that has dropped significantly to below $1,000 by 2020.[43] So today, almost anyone can do it. Here's how it works:

Our DNA is read through a process called genotyping that determines the sequence of the nucleotides (A, T, C, and G) in a DNA strand. DNA sequencing allows scientists to differentiate and compare the regular versions for the gene variants and mutations. They can then compare all the genomes that have been sequenced to identify the similarities and differences. That can help them figure out the chances of the disease developing, optimize treatment protocols, and most importantly, implement prevention methods. We may all have similar features, but we are all unique at the genetic level.

FUN FACT:

Think of your DNA raw data like your fingerprint. One day, it might become linked to your cellphone and email address, so if you have a mutation linked to certain diseases, you might get spammed with emails and calls for supplements to combat that condition.

Genomic tests are typically offered either as a panel of targeted genes or a full-range gene sequencing performed by specialized CLIA labs. Most tests require either:

- A saliva sample.
- A swab from inside your cheek, known as a buccal smear.
- A blood test.

There are three basic methods of attaining genetic data and reading an organism's genome.

1. GENOTYPING USING SNPs

This is the most common and the least expensive option. It's the method used when you sign up for 23&Me or Ancestry.com. It's a screening process where scientists study the differences in the genotype of an individual. It uses DNA sequencing and compares it to a different sequence for reference. It looks for common DNA different variants or SNPs. If you were to change the "D" in the word "Dog" to an "L," youwould change the meaning of the word, right? The same is true when a single nucleotide changes. It can alter the functioning of a gene and have significant consequences. SNPs help discover any mutations or variations of the genes that can aid with the prevention, diagnosis, and specific treatment of a disease.

This method is good for learning about single-gene traits and common conditions and diseases such as the MC1R gene (red hair), CFTR gene (cystic fibrosis), and BRCA1 and BRCA2 genes (breast cancer). It's less ideal for identifying complex diseases such as type 2 diabetes and Alzheimer's disease. However, more research is being conducted, and as more genomes are sequenced, the outcome of the tests for complex diseases will improve.

This is the most common and affordable method, and one that you can administer on your own without the supervision of a practitioner. The next section provides a list of some popular and reliable companies who offer this service.

2. WHOLE-EXOME SEQUENCING

This method looks at more of the DNA than the first method and is more involved and more expensive because of that. Exons are a portion of our DNA that carry instructions on making proteins, but they only account for around 1 percent of the entire genome.[44] The group of exons in a genome is called the exome, and most of the genetic mutations that cause disease occur in the exome. Exome sequencing is thought to be an efficient method to identify possible disease-causing mutations. Right now, the cost is in the thousands, but prices are dropping as the demand increases and more companies offer these services. As mentioned, this test would be conducted through a practitioner since a tissue sample is required.

3. WHOLE-GENOME SEQUENCING (WGS)

This is the most thorough and comprehensive of all the methods. It's an extensive analysis of your genes, and it's also the most expensive. This gets everything—junk DNA and all. The problem is that we still don't understand what some of the material gathered with this test means, because there hasn't been enough data accumulated to recognize any patterns.

This method is ideal for the discovery of novel driver mutations. If I'm working with a patient who has been diagnosed with cancer, I recommend these last two methods because most cancers appear on the exome. Illumina is a great company that provides this service, and they have been involved since the Human Genome Project. Again, the practitioner would be the one who would walk you through this process. It wouldn't be something you would do on your own.

FUN FACT:

For one person to have their whole genome read, it used to cost over $100,000; but today you can find companies that will do it for around $3,000. That's how quickly the technology is advancing.

GETTING YOUR DNA RAW DATA FROM HOME

You have plenty of options when it comes to having your genome read. Here is a list of companies for you to consider to find the best fit for you.

Genotyping Using SNPs:

- 23andMe
- AncestryDNA
- Illumina
- Oxford Nanopore
- Sophia Genetics
- Veritas Genetics
- Family Tree DNA
- Pathway
- Helix
- MyHeritage
- LivingDNA
- Genomelink
- Promethease
- GEDmatch
- MyTrue Ancestry
- LivingDNA
- African Ancestry

- Nebula Genomics
- SelfDecode
- Xcode Life
- Genopalate
- Athletigen
- FitnessGenes
- Vitagene
- DNAFit
- Sano Genetics
- Luna DNA
- Sequencing.com
- Gene Plaza
- AxGen

Exome Sequencing:

- Genos
- BGI
- Omega
- 14 Labs
- Gene-by-Gene

Whole Genome Sequencing

- Nebula Genomics
- Veritas Genetics
- BGI-CGI-MGI
- Dante Labs
- Dante Labs GenomeZ
- Genomics Personalize Health
- Macrogen
- MapMyGenome
- Novogene
- SureGenomics
- Gene-by-Gene
- Illumina UYG

- Illumina Clinical
- Partners LMM
- GeneDx
- Cloud Health

Cancer Exome or Genome Sequencing

- Illumina
- Mayo Clinic
- Alacris
- Foundation Medicine

When I first started, 23&Me was the only company that provided this service. Now, so many people are interested in learning about their heritage and DNA that more and more of these companies are popping up. By the start of 2019, more than 26 million people had uploaded their data to the various databases, and that number is predicted to reach 100 million by 2025.[45] Imagine how much data there will be to study and how much more we will know about the human genome in only a few years.

I don't prefer one company over another, but I recommend that people go with the companies that provide you with your DNA raw data, such as 23andMe and Ancestry.com. Those seem to be the most popular options. They provide you with your raw data (that you then upload to the services and sites listed in the next section for it to be interpreted), while a service like PathwayFit is different. They don't give you your raw data but interpret it for you by making supplement, nutrition, and exercise recommendations. This is why knowledge and research are essential, so you can find the service that best fits your needs.

Once you have your raw data, you don't need to ever take the test again. You only need to run your genetic profile once because your genes don't change over time. Unless you were to utilize CRISPR/Cas-9 technology to cut and reconnect your genes, the results you receive are permanent. They are like your fingerprints. How they are expressed (turned on or off) can change, but that information will NOT show up in a genetic profile. The test can tell you if you have a certain mutation or are susceptible to a disease, but you will have to rely on other symptoms to determine if that gene has been expressed or not.

FUN FACT:

If you're undecided and can't think of ideas for holiday, birthday gifts or special occasions consider one of these tests. They can provide many random facts that make for a good dinner conversation.

YOU HAVE THE RESULTS, NOW WHAT?

It depends on what company you chose to conduct your genetic test, but some companies have their own labs to analyze the data. Both 23&Me and Ancestry allow you to keep that raw data. What you do with it depends on what you're trying to achieve and what you want to learn. Here are some options:

- SNPedia: This is a worldwide database that scientists use to compile data, recognize trends, and advance their understanding of genomics. You can upload your data, and it will tell you what a particular gene does, but it won't tell you how to take care of the potential issue that might arise through nutrition and supplementation. You can type in various SNPs and genes, and you will be provided with pages and information that can get overly scientific at times. Keep in mind that the data from 23andMe is anonymously reported to SNPedia.

- Prometheus: This is a pay site that can thoroughly explain what your specific gene mutations mean. It's a beautiful research website that allows you to upload your raw data. They share their data with 23&Me and SNPedia as well. This is where I get a lot of my information, and it has two different sections for disease—one for medical diseases and the other for medical diseases based on the genome, to see what you are genetically predisposed to. If you know how to navigate their systems, it can tell you the percentage of heart disease in your family. It details studies that were conducted, and all of the relevant information related to that study. This site is personalized, but it's also thorough, so the science and explanation can get complicated.

- GeneCards: This is another amazing site similar to SNPedia that provides a lot of information about what your raw data really means.

- Knowyourgenetics.com: This is a database compiled by the NRI (Neurological Research Institute) run by Dr. Amy Yasko. This is a great site with some excellent information, and a lot of supplement recommendations.

- Genetic Genie: This is a totally free site specific to the Cytochrome P450 pathway (which we will discuss in the next chapter) that allows you to update your raw data and learn your detox pathways. Think of it this way: There are 50 or 60 genes linked to the Cytochrome P40 pathway, which is the primary pathway involved in liver detoxification. It's how your body gets rid of toxins. Food and supplements also have to go through the liver (pretty much everything has to go through the liver), so it can be helpful to know if any of those genes have a mutation that could impair that pathway or how you process certain food, supplements, or drugs. We've learned so much since I first started incorporating genomics into my practice, that the size of the specialized report Genetic Genie provides has doubled in that time.

- AxGen: This is a company founded by Dr. Stuart Kim that we will discuss in more detail when we get to fitness and exercise, because that's their specialty. Their services are offered to everyone, but they specialize in athletes. That means professional athletes, weekend warriors, and even the parents of young kids playing sports can all benefit. You can upload your raw data (or provide a cheek swab to get genotyped), and they can provide the necessary training recommendations to maximize the potential of your genes while avoiding injuries you might be genetically susceptible to.

Genome sequencing is becoming a powerful and useful tool in medicine, molecular biology, evolutionary biology, forensics, ecology, agriculture, and virology. The technological advancements, coupled with the rapid decrease in cost, make this a rapidly growing field. Hundreds of thousands of people have had their genome analyzed, and as more people have the test done, it creates more data to study. With data regularly being uploaded to SNPedia and these various worldwide databases, scientists can study and analyze that data to recognize patterns. This helps clinicians identify more people with a predisposition to common illnesses, find answers for how to treat rare diseases, and personalize medicine according to the individual genome.

When everyone shares their information, this global effort can lead to faster advancements in the future. However, now that there is more data and more companies in control of that data, there are some legal challenges that make data sharing more difficult.[46] That can be expected because this is such a new science, but those at the forefront of the industry know the incredible benefits of sharing data, so I'm confident the situation will be improved in years to come.

Despite the hurdles, these are all great references that are used extensively when it comes to mapping diseases. When uploading your raw data, you aren't only helping yourself; you are helping each other because you're adding more data to the system. I witnessed this first-hand when treating a patient with a rare type of cancer. For cancer patients, their raw data is uploaded into the database at the Cancer Genome Atlas Program. This can aid in treatment and can help us see the pathway that a particular cancer prefers. When I first started treating my patient in 2019, I couldn't find a single study relating to her specific form of cancer. But the following year there were 206 studies, 50 of which proved helpful in treating her cancer. We could see the pathway and determine which type of chemotherapy and radiation worked best, while coming up with a more personalized supplement and nutrition program. That's why I like to think of genomics as the gift that keeps on giving.

FUN FACT:

Do you remember how they finally caught the Golden State Killer in 2018? It was through DNA, but more specifically, it was through an online service called GEDmatch, which is a database compatible with different testing companies like 23andMe and Ancestry.com, so customers can upload their data. Authorities were able to link the previously unidentified DNA of the killer to that of a relative in the system.

IS MY RAW DATA SAFE?

As DNA testing and sites like 23&Me have become more popular, there is also more talk about privacy concerns and if the raw data accumulated by these companies is safe.

The simple answer is "yes." Your raw data is safe, but there is still a room for improvement, and a lot that needs to be figured out. This is a brand-new science, so when it comes to regulations and legalities, we are in uncharted territory and learning as we go. Just like the authorities need a court order to obtain a search warrant for your home, the same is true for your DNA. Think about how people were once afraid to use their credit cards when making purchases online due to security issues and fraud. Since then, steps have been taken to not only make online purchases safer than ever but to make them the preferred way of shopping. In time, we should expect the same type of security when it comes to protecting our raw data and downloading it to various sites online. Strides are already being made. Back in 2008, Congress signed the GINA Act (the Genetic Information Nondiscrimination Act), which prevents genetic discrimination. There is protection at the federal level, but a lot also depends on where in the country you live, because some states have more protection than others.

FUN FACT:
Our DNA would fill up 100 encyclopedia volumes.

CHAPTER 4:

_____

BEFORE YOU DO ANYTHING, DETOX YOUR SYSTEM

You have your raw data, but before you change your diet, purchase supplements, or even begin to think about how to maximize your genes' efficiency, you want to reset your system, and the best way to do that is through a detox. It's the very first thing I do with most of my patients, unless they are suffering from certain underlying conditions such as liver issues, kidney concerns, immunocompromised conditions or gut inflammation that require us to first address those issues.

Why a detox? Because your gut is your connection to the outside world. Everything you eat, drink, and ingest has to be processed through your gut, blood vessels, liver, and kidneys, so if toxins and inflammation are impeding your digestion and clogging up your system, you won't be able to absorb nutrients or supplements properly. Not only can a detox improve your gut health, impact your genome, and influence which genes are turned on and off, but it's a great way to get healthier and cleanse your entire system.

TOXINS ARE EVERYWHERE!

The environment is full of toxins that we're exposed to every day through the food we eat, our environment, the drugs we take (prescription and recreational), and even the products we use. There is no avoiding it. Your computer, and most of the perfumes, deodorants, and laundry detergents on the market, have toxins. Some are more harmful than others, but they are still contaminants, unless you use natural products. Short of living your life in a bubble, it's virtually impossible not to be exposed to any toxins.

We've been aware of toxins for a very long time. The ancient Romans knew the danger of metals such as mercury, lead, and arsenic. In her 1962 book *Silent Spring*, marine biologist Rachel Carson created public awareness of how industrial chemicals could harm humans after studying the effect of the pesticide DDT on various birds. Why do you think smokestacks are built so high? It's so they can keep the toxins as far above the ground and away from the people as possible.

There are over 100,000 different chemicals available for commercial use, and we still don't completely understand all of the effects they can have on our bodies. And not only are the living susceptible but so are the unborn, as toxins can be passed from mother to child. We are exposed to these toxins through four main pathways: skin, lungs, ingestion, and injection.

Believe it or not, our greatest toxin exposure is by far from what we put into our bodies—specifically food, water, and drugs.[47] In the United States alone, close to 4,000 additives are allowed in foods and are commonly divided into the following categories:

- Preservatives (BHT, BHA, sulfite, nitrogen oxide)
- Food colorings (FD&C yellow #5)
- Sweeteners (aspartame)
- Stimulants (caffeine)
- Flavor enhancers (MSG)[48]

Over time, these toxins can build up and be stored in the body. When that happens, they primarily affect three main organs and six systems:

ORGANS

- Liver: Filters toxins out of the blood, so they can be eliminated through urine or stool.
- Kidneys: Provide a route for toxins to be eliminated through urine.
- Intestines: Where toxins can build up and ultimately leak into the bloodstream.

SYSTEMS

- Integumentary/Exocrine system aka skin, hair, and nails.
- Digestive system which includes the mouth, esophagus, stomach, pancreas, liver, gallbladder, small intestine, appendix, large intestine, and anus.
- Urinary system and its components of kidneys, ureters, bladder, and urethra.
- Lymphatic and Immune System which includes the white blood cells, antibodies, spleen, tonsils and adenoids, thymus gland, lymph fluid and lymph vessels, nodes, and glands.
- Respiratory System and its components of nose, skull, throat, windpipe, lungs, diaphragm, and respiratory muscles.
- Endocrine system aka hormone regulation which includes parts of the brain, the thyroid gland, parathyroids, adrenals, the ovaries and the testes.

As mentioned earlier we have 11 body systems and even though these systems are described as separate entities for anatomical purposes, each body system depends on each other for physical, physiological and nutritional support. Eventually, if toxins are not addressed they have the potential to affect all of our 11 systems.

The body does have natural defenses in the form of membrane barriers, enzymes, and antioxidants to eliminate these toxins through:

- Urine
- Breath
- Sweat
- Feces
- Saliva

However, your body can't get rid of them all, especially if your organ-systems are compromised, so toxins build up over time and place a burden on your detox organs and lymphatic system. But don't forget that no two people are the same. Your level of susceptibility to certain toxins depends on your genome, age, overall health, and any prior conditions; but even the healthiest individual has toxins in their system. I've never tested a patient who didn't have toxins. It's unavoidable.

FUN FACT:

Our liver regulates our hormones, and if imbalanced can cause estrogen to accumulate, leading to premenstrual syndrome, polycystic ovarian syndrome, and even some cancers.[49]

THE MAIN CULPRITS

Don't assume that just because toxins are referred to as "environmental" that they are harmless. They can still have an impact in low doses and continue to accumulate in your body. Your exposure depends on conditions that vary from lifestyle to where you live. However, I have noticed patterns, and some toxins are much more common than others. One of the main factors is where people live. My patients who live by the beach tend to have more toxicity from plastic.

These are the four most common toxins that I've found in my patients:

1. ALUMINUM: Bacteria can hold onto aluminum, which is also known to inhibit glutamate dehydrogenase, and increased glutamate can lead to cell death and impair brain function in the long term.[50] Aluminum also interferes with the production of BH4, which can affect levels of serotonin and dopamine.

Sources: Believe it or not, the most common source of aluminum is in the products we use every day. Deodorant is loaded with aluminum. Are you used to cooking or storing your food in aluminum foil? There is another source. Even the fillings in your teeth and some of your silverware at home might contain aluminum.

2. MERCURY: Mercury can inhibit the activity of glutamate synthase. Under ideal conditions, glutamine, glutamate, GABA, and alpha-ketoglutarate can interconvert to form the intermediates that the body requires at any given time. Mercury can also inhibit the MTRR pathway, and can cause anemia and the inability to make groups that are needed for B12 synthesis. Mercury exposure can lead to reduced sensory abilities (such as taste, touch, vision, and hearing), fatigue, irritability, excitability, tremors, hypertension, neuromuscular disorders, and an increased risk of cardiovascular disease.[51] Some early symptoms include loss of appetite, depression, emotional instability, and decreased sense of touch, hearing, and vision.

Sources: Mercury can be found in fish (salmon, tuna), skin-lightening agents, instruments (like thermometers, batteries), and dental fillings.

3. LEAD: This toxin can deposit itself in bone and replace the calcium in bone while also affecting ATP, which is a stored form of energy. ATP is a molecule in the mitochondria, which is the powerhouse of the cell. Lead can decrease this, ultimately leading to a reduction of energy. The presence of lead negatively impacts both sodium and potassium levels. Lead excretion can cause pica, teeth grinding, and signs of aggression, in addition to depressing immune system function, anemia, headache, fatigue, weight loss, hypertension, kidney disease, and increased tooth decay. Cognition and mental development can be significantly impacted by exposure to lead.

Sources: Women's beauty products, particularly lipstick, are loaded with lead. Some fertilizers, newsprint, and candles contain lead. Lead is also a gasoline additive that was used in paint before 1982. The solder in plumbing contains lead, so your exposure might be higher if you are in these environments. Thankfully, our knowledge about the dangers of lead have grown over the years because it was often found in everyday items. Many believe that Queen

Elizabeth I became ill and died from blood poisoning that was a result of the lead-based makeup that was popular in the era.

4. CADMIUM: This is another toxin that's very common and difficult for the body to eliminate on its own. You probably haven't heard of it because it's not nearly as well-known as the first three, but it can do some damage. It's a chemical element mostly found in zinc ores and byproducts. Long-term exposure can result in the loss of smell, anemia, dry skin, hair loss, hypertension, and kidney problems.

Sources: The primary way cadmium gets into our bodies is through our food sources that come from the ground, because cadmium is often present in the soil. It can also be found in shellfish and cigarette smoke.

THE IMPACT

The skin is the largest organ in the body, so it will absorb the chemicals in the products that you put on it. Once these toxins accumulate, it's like a domino effect. Overexposure typically impacts brain function, leading to fogginess, fatigue, headache, and lack of concentration. This can lead to thyroid and hormonal issues. When these toxins are removed after the detox, people definitely see improved brain function and energy level.

FUN FACT:

Our liver cleanses our blood 24 hours a day, 7 days a week, 365 days a year. It filters nearly 380 liters of blood every day to remove a number of micro-organisms such as bacteria, fungi, viruses, and parasites from our bloodstream.[52]

HEAVY METALS & NON-HEAVY METALS

Just to give you an idea of what you might be exposed to, here is list of common heavy metals:

Arsenic

Lead

Mercury

Cadmium

Chromium

Beryllium

Cobalt

Nickel

Zinc

Copper

Thorium

Thallium

Barium

Cesium

Manganese

Selenium

Bismuth

Vanadium

Silver

Antimony

Platinum

Tungsten

Tin

Uranium

Gold

Tellurium

Germanium

Titanium

Gadolinium

These are non-environmental, non-heavy-metal pollutants:

Phthalates

Vinyl chloride

Benzene

Pyrethrins

Xylenes

Styrene

Organophosphates

MTBE and ETBE

2,4 Dicholorophenoxyacetic (2,4-D)

Diphenyl phosphate

Acrylamide

Perchlorate

1,3 Butadiene

Propylene oxide

1-Bromopropane

Ethylene oxide

Acrylonitrile

Acrolein

These metals can attach to your DNA and do damage by changing that DNA. That can be linked to the following conditions, which is why the detox is so important, and can be such a major step in the right direction because it helps us avoid developing some of these conditions before they become an issue.

Alzheimer's disease

Amyotrophic lacteroclerosis (ALS)

Anorexia nervosa

Anxiety disorder

Apraxia

Arthritis

Asthma

Attention deficit disorder (ADD)

Attention deficit with hyperactivity (ADHD)

Autism

Autoimmune disorders

Bipolar disorder

Cancer

Cerebral palsy

Chronic fatigue syndrome

Crohn's disease

Depression

Developmental disorder

Down syndrome

Epilepsy

Failure to thrive

Fibromyalgia

Genetic diseases

Irritable bowel syndrome

Learning disability

Mitochondria disorder

Multiple sclerosis

Obsessive-compulsive disorder (OCD)

Occupational exposures

Parkinson's disease

Peripheral neuropathy

Schizophrenia

Seizure disorders

Systemic lupus erythematosus

Tic disorders

Tourette syndrome

Ulcerative colitis

CHANGES YOU CAN MAKE TODAY

Detox may be the best way to remove those stubborn toxins that can remain in the body for extended periods, but it's better to prevent them from entering the body at all because the body doesn't know what to do with them. Certain levels are considered normal, but in my opinion, you should strive to have no aluminum, mercury, lead, or cadmium in the body. In part, this is impossible, because toxins will inevitably enter your body, but you can do things to prevent the level of toxins you are exposed to. Simply being more aware of how toxins get into your system can help you avoid them in the future; but there are some simple changes you can immediately make today that will limit your exposure. Little changes in your lifestyle can make a big difference over time.

*ORGANICS: If it's possible and within your budget, see if you can switch to natural or organic household items and food products. Instead of aluminum foil, try using parchment paper. Look for a natural deodorant that doesn't contain any aluminum. When you buy fruits and vegetables, try to buy organic to avoid chemicals and pesticides. The U.S. Department of Agriculture found that even after washing (and sometimes even after peeling), the following fruits and vegetables still contained a high pesticide residue, so consider always buying organic versions of these specific fruits and vegetables:[53]

1. Strawberries

2. Apples

3. Nectarines

4. Peaches

5. Celery

6. Grapes

7. Cherries

8. Spinach

9. Tomatoes

10. Sweet bell peppers

11. Cherry tomatoes

12. Cucumbers

The following foods were shown to have less pesticide residue, so if you opt not to buy organic, it's best to do it with these fruits and vegetables.

1. Avocados

2. Sweet corn

3. Pineapples

4. Cabbage

5. Sweet peas (frozen)

6. Onions

7. Asparagus

8. Mangos

9. Papayas

10. Kiwi

11. Eggplant

12. Honeydew melon

13. Grapefruit

14. Cantaloupe

15. Cauliflower

*PLASTICS: In general, you want to avoid all plastics. In my house, we don't use plastics at all and have replaced everything plastic with glass. I also realize that this isn't always possible, especially for families with kids, so you want to make sure you're using the safest plastics possible. To be sure, look at the bottom of the actual container. Next to the triangle, you should find a number that signifies the material in that plastic. Numbers 2, 4, and 5 are considered safe. Numbers 1, 3, 6, and 7 are the most harmful and contain known carcinogens.

*WATER FILTERS: This depends on your budget. I've had some clients pay tens of thousands of dollars to install water purification systems throughout the entire house. You can also find a basic filter for $50 that you can put on your faucet and showerhead, to purify the water in your home. If you're unsure about the quality of your drinking water, Doctor's Data offers a Comprehensive Drinking Water Analysis test that is a great and inexpensive way to analyze the water in your home.[54]

*AIR FILTERS: This also depends on your budget. Short of installing a house-wide system, you can buy an affordable portable air filter that can protect you from molds and other toxins that can affect your DNA. If someone has respiratory issues, a weak immune system, or is going through chemotherapy, they could benefit from a sterile environment. In some cases, I recommend oxygen therapy because oxygen equals life.

I always want to be thorough and measure these specific toxins in my patients, so I know exactly what area to target. These tests are conducted by taking samples of hair, blood, or urine. Blood and urine samples are good for recent exposure to contaminants, while hair samples prove more long-term exposure. Here is a list of reliable toxic metal and toxic non-metal lab tests:

- Doctor's Data: Comprehensive Blood Elements
- Doctor's Data: Hair Elements
- Genova Diagnostics: Toxic Exposure Test
- Genova Diagnostics: Nutrient & Toxic Elements—Whole Blood
- Genova Diagnostics: Toxic Metals—Whole Blood
- The Great Plains Laboratory - MycoTOX Profile (Mold Exposure)
- Genova Diagnostics: Oxidative Stress Analysis 2.0 (blood and urine)
- The Great Plains Laboratory—GPL—TOX Profile—Toxic Non-Metal Chemicals
- The Great Plains Laboratory—Glyphosate (herbicide)
- US BioTek Laboratories—Environmental Pollutant Profile
- Real Time Laboratories—Environmental Mold and Mycotoxin Assessment
- Microbiology DX—MARCoNS and Mold Culture with Identification

CLEARING PATHWAYS

There are all different types of pathways in the body.

The process in which DNA makes cells, cells make tissues, tissues make organs, and organs make systems all follow a pathway. The way cancer develops in the body follows a pathway. The way the body produces testosterone or estrogen follows a pathway. Even methylation follows a pathway.

One of the biggest and most significant pathways in the body is the Cytochrome P450 pathway. It's a family of over 50 enzymes, six of which metabolize 90 percent of drugs, with the two most significant enzymes being CYP3A4 and CYP2D6.[55] It's located in the liver, so everything we digest (food, supplements, and medication) has to pass through it, which is what makes this pathway particularly important.

We know about these pathways because every time something happens in your body, it leaves a trace. We can detect if something is wrong or not working correctly by following the traces along these various pathways. Let's say there is some metal toxicity attached to a liver cell or a brain cell that negatively impacts the way that gene functions.

The detox works as a scavenger to remove those metals and those reactive oxygen species (ROS), which are the byproducts of food and environmental toxins that can harm your DNA. In doing so, it clears these pathways so the body can function better.

DETOX OPTIONS

You have a lot of options when it comes to detox programs, but the one I personally use and recommend to my patients is by Metagenics. I don't work for Metagenics or have any affiliation with the company, but it's the one that I believe to be the most effective. If you chose to go this route, you have two options:

- 10-day detox
- 28-day detox

As expected, the 28-day version is mild but longer, while the 10-day is more intense but shorter. No matter which option you chose, you get a similar effect. I tend to favor the 28-day detox because the longer timeframe helps to establish healthier eating patterns. The programs are each very extensive and involve a combination of diet recommendations, nutritional shakes, vitamins, and supplements. Both detox programs are very similar to the more popular elimination diets and focus on many of the same basic principles:

- Eliminate dairy and milk in favor of substitutes like almond, coconut, or oat milk.
- Avoid meat in favor of free-range, cold-water fish.
- Eliminate gluten and grain in favor of non-gluten grains like brown rice, millet, oats, and quinoa.
- Drink two quarts of filtered water daily.
- Avoid alcohol and caffeine.
- Avoid citrus in favor of whole fruits and raw, steamed, sautéed vegetables.
- Avoid soybean products in favor of dried beans, split peas, and legumes.
- Avoid butter, margarine, salad dressings, mayonnaise, and processed oils in favor of cold-pressed olive and flaxseed oils.

To get a more comprehensive feel for what's involved in the Metagenics detox and how it works, you can look at the actual programs, which I have included for you in the Appendix. For the most part, I recommend that my patients follow the program exactly as laid out, but I often do make one modification. They allow white rice, but because of its high glycemic index, I recommend only eating brown rice or quinoa.

If you don't feel like the Metagenics program is a good fit for you, here is a list of other companies that offer quality detox programs:

- Orthomolecular Products—Core Restore 7-Day Kit
  ▷ https://www.orthomolecularproducts.com/
- Pure Encapsulations—Detox Program
  ▷ https://www.pureencapsulations.com/media/brch_Detox.pdf
- Vital Nutrients—Comprehensive Detox Kit
  ▷ https://www.vitalnutrients.net/detox-kit.html
- Standard Process—Detox Balance Program
  ▷ https://www.standardprocess.com/programs/
    detox-cleanse-supplements

FUN FACT:

The inclusion of flaxseeds, pumpkin seeds, walnuts, water, vegetables, and fruits in our diet can aid the skin during the detoxification process.[56]

HOW THE DETOX WORKS

There are three phases to the detox:

I: Biotransformation.

II: Conjugation

III: Elimination

One of the primary goals is to remove toxins that can't otherwise be secreted by the body, to improve organ function and prevent certain genes from being expressed. How does that occur? It changes the state of the toxins.

To put it simply, there are two types of toxins:

- Fat-soluble toxins
- Water-soluble toxins

Fat-soluble toxins are the ones with the most damaging health effects, and can remain in the body for years because they are harbored in the fatty tissues. Water-soluble toxins are less harmful and more easily removed from the body naturally. This is what occurs during the first stage of biotransformation. During the second phase, conjugation, fat-soluble toxins are converted to water-soluble toxins so they can be removed from the body before they can enter the bloodstream. The higher a person's body fat, the more potential toxins they have, and the more difficult they are to remove, which is one of the reasons why overweight individuals are susceptible to so many different acute and chronic conditions.

After detox, only a small amount of toxins and metals make their way through the liver, kidneys, intestines, and ultimately into the bloodstream. The organs aren't overburdened and are better able to function correctly.

BE READY TO CHANGE YOUR DIET

When I first started using Metagenics products back in 1998, they only had one option, and it was a 28-day cleanse. The diet consisted primarily of shakes. I definitely felt the benefits, but it wasn't always easy to incorporate the program into my every-day life. Thankfully, over the past 22 years, they've modified and improved the program significantly. There is more variety now, and it's much easier to work the program without completely altering the way you eat and live.

Despite the improvements, YOU WILL have to make changes to your diet. Remember, this isn't a restrictive diet. You aren't going to starve yourself or be on a liquid diet, but as your food intake decreases and your food choices get more refined, the amount of cleanse shakes you drink will increase. You do have to modify what you eat because the program is:

Gluten-free

Sugar-free

Dairy-free

Alcohol-free

Caffeine-free

In my experience, there are four things that my patients find the most challenging to remove from their diet during the detox.

1. SUGAR: Too much sugar in your diet can lead to weight gain, and an increased chance of developing heart disease, type 2 diabetes, cancer, and a number of other diseases. Sugar can lead to cellular aging, while draining your energy.

2. CAFFEINE: Fermented teas are okay to consume, but caffeine is the most common stimulant, and most people consume caffeine in coffee and energy drinks. It can be harmless in small doses, but can cause anxiety, insomnia, headaches, digestive problems, and even high blood pressure. Too much caffeine can prevent the absorption of certain vitamins and minerals.

3. SALT: High sodium intake can lead to high blood pressure. Most commercial foods have large amounts of hidden sodium. Foods high in salt include salted nuts, canned beans, frozen food, and smoked meats.

4. ALCOHOL: The harmful effects of alcohol are well-known. Alcohol dehydrogenase 1C (ADH1C) metabolizes alcohol, creating acetaldehyde, a toxic substance responsible for hangovers.

COMMIT YOURSELF

Everyone is different, and how easily you can incorporate the detox depends on your lifestyle. Those with healthier eating habits who exercise regularly usually have an easier time adapting. However, even the healthiest patients of mine still have to make a change, because there are aspects of their everyday life that are disrupted during the detox. If you haven't completed a detox before, the first time around can be challenging; but the better prepared you are for potential disruptions, the easier it will be for you to adapt.

Often, it's the little things that can trip people up. Are you a coffee drinker? Well, you can't drink coffee when detoxing. Do you usually have a beer or a glass of wine after work or with dinner? That has to stop during the detox. Depending on how much caffeine and alcohol you typically ingest, you might experience headaches and withdrawal for a couple of days. What's funny is that I've had a few clients tell me that before they went on the detox, they would have three or four glasses of wine before feeling the effect; but after detox, all they needed was half a glass. That's what cleansing your liver and resetting your system can do.

Because of the potential impact of those little changes, the detox starts slow, and you ease your way into it. I've known patients who have hidden food under the bed and talked themselves into cheating. Unfortunately, those patients never experience the full benefit.

I may have done multiple detoxes, and I have gotten used to it, but that doesn't mean I think it's easy. I know that it can be challenging at times. That's why I have my patients come into the office every week to discuss their challenges. When I chart their progress, it motivates them and gets them excited; but it's also a way to hold them accountable. I try to reiterate the importance of what they're doing while showing them how it will benefit their long-term health. Some patients need that boost more than others, but no matter your situation or where you're starting from, the biggest motivator is the way you feel. When you begin to feel better, that is a great natural way to reinforce these new habits and behaviors, because when you change your habits, you change your life. For patients that can't come to the office during detox, keeping a detox journal describing your experiences and feelings always helps.

In the end, it comes down to the will of the person and how much the detox is out of their comfort zone. It may be hard, but it's worth it. This process does require change, because we are creatures of habit and change can be difficult, but as the great Einstein said, "The definition of insanity is doing the same thing and expecting different results." The way I see it, it always comes back to habits. Good or bad, your habits will determine your level of success. "Your current habits are perfectly designed to deliver your current result." That's one of my favorite quotes by James Clear. For my patients who are struggling, I recommend they read the classic book, *The 7 Habits of Highly Effective People* by Stephen Covey, a copy of which I keep under the desk; and *The Four Agreements by* Don Miquel Ruiz. But all change comes from within and seeing the detox through until the end is half the battle. I don't know of a single person who has stuck with it and didn't notice the positive effect on their overall health and well-being.

FUN FACT:

Toxins may be the reason why you wake up at unusual hours during the night, since the liver is most active at night.[57]

LONG-TERM BENEFITS

Not only does the detox cleanse your system, but there are a host of ancillary benefits that can improve your overall health. Many patients notice a change in their skin—even my staff can notice how they have more of a vibrant, youthful glow. The improvement isn't just external but internal as well, as they think better, manage stress better, and aren't feeling as fatigued or tired. I've seen clients who have made lifelong changes after completing the detox because the process gave them a different perspective. They changed the way they thought about food, so they naturally started making healthier choices. These are the most common life changes I've witnessed:

Weight Loss

This is a big one, as you can imagine. So many people want to lose weight, and this is an excellent way to do it because one benefit of the detox is that it can help you shed pounds, even if that isn't your main goal. That's why I call weight loss a side effect of the detox. When you have three shakes a day, it fills you up, so you eat less food, and you're eating healthy food. This isn't a restrictive diet, so the goal isn't weight loss, but I don't remember having a client who didn't lose weight. On average, most of my clients lose between 5 and 10 pounds when on the 28-day detox. The losses are less on the 10-day detox, but still noticeable. That alone is worth it for many. It can also improve your overall well-being while combating fatigue and digestive issues.

Creating Healthy Habits

Humans are creatures of habit. That works both for us and against us. Some of those habits are good, and others are not, but the detox can help you create more healthy habits. How is that possible? Think of it like this: it is possible to change a habit in under 30 days. If you're used to eating pizza, candy, and fast food, and drinking diet soda—which is common and something we're all guilty of at times—after the detox, you might not crave the same foods because your taste buds can change. Yes, our taste buds can change in as little as 21 days.[58] Start eating food that is better for you, and it can grow on you. I've had clients who were used to eating sweets before the detox try to eat a candy bar after the detox and tell me they could barely get through two bites. In fact, they couldn't believe how they had been eating junk food for so long.

Even though the 10-day detox and the 28-day detox serve the same function, I have noticed that the 28-day detox is more likely to lead to significant change. The reason is that it's more of a sacrifice, and you have to sustain it longer, so you strengthen new good habits while further removing yourself from old bad ones.

Learning How to Read Labels

If you were one of those people who never paid much attention to the ingredients in the food you bought before the detox, that will probably change. The reason is that you will have to learn how to shop. By default, the detox will give you a crash course in nutrition and nutrients. That first week can be frustrating and overwhelming because it might seem like you're spending so much time at the grocery store, but you will quickly learn to recognize carcinogens and know what foods to avoid. Soon, that will become a habit, and you will learn what's healthy and where to go to find it.

Reduce the Need for Medication

This is absolutely something you need to consult with your doctor before doing, but I've had patients who have been able to lower the dosage on the medication they've taken while some have been able to get off certain medications altogether.

Tim was a patient of mine who was reluctant to try something alternative, as he had only been exposed to mainstream medicine. Once he started to experience horrible side effects from the statin medication he was taking for his high cholesterol, he finally came in. The first thing we did was modify the supportive detox to last the entire 40 days of Lent, as it was his yearly practice to give something up. It worked great. His cholesterol levels immediately dropped 48 points, and he lost 18 pounds. We then did a genomic analysis, and low and behold, he had a mutation that impacted how his body processed statin medication. I spoke with his doctor, and we consulted the FDA recommendation for dosage, but since Tim already decreased his cholesterol by 48 points, his doctor put him on observation. That was five years ago. He stuck to his diet, does a yearly 28-day Metagenics detox, maintained a healthy weight, and his cholesterol still remains normal without ever having to go back on the medication.

Improve Some Pre-Existing Conditions

Don't get me wrong. This isn't a miracle cure, but losing weight, getting healthier, and cleansing your system can help alleviate symptoms and the need for some medication. For my patients with high cholesterol, most of them lost 30 points right off the bat. The most I've ever seen a patient lose is 48, but that was my patient who modified the detox to last all 40 days of Lent. But even the 10-day detox will reset your system and possibly lower the need for statin medication in some cases. Please remember that before you adjust any medication, you must consult with your doctor. That isn't anything you want to do without medical supervision.

THE IMPORTANCE OF A HEALTHY MICROBIOME

Microbes are everywhere—inside our bodies and out. When we're born, billions of bacteria cover our bodies as we pass through the birth canal, but this isn't a bad thing. Bacteria don't just cause disease; they can help us and influence our overall health, too. Every human has their own unique microbiome made up of various forms of fungus, bacteria, viruses, and organisms—some work against our body to do us harm, and some work with our body to keep us healthy. While 99.9 percent of our genome may be the same, everyone has a very different microbiome, and we share only 5 percent of the same microbial DNA.[59]

Research continues to evolve, but as of right now, the microbial cells in our bodies outnumber the human cells by about ten to one. This is nothing new. These microbes have been on earth for three billion years. Our organs even evolved to house these microbes. It almost seems like they are the host, and we are visitors in their world. Right when babies are born, their gut microbiome resembles their mother's vaginal microbiome. It develops significantly during the first year of life, and it's very dependent on the environment.

For example, infants fed breast milk have a different microbiome than those fed formula.

By the time a child reaches the age of three, their microbiome begins to resemble that of an adult. As we continue to age, environment, diet, sleep, fitness, stress, and exposure to toxins all impact our microbiome. Where we live (rural or urban), the number of siblings we have, and even our pets can impact our microbiome. Even the chemicals found in the house can have an impact on the microbiome of children.[60] It's a fascinating topic. Not only does vitamin B come from gut microbes, and the skin microbiome can affect our attractiveness to mosquitos, but there were even new bacterial strains found aboard the International Space Station.[61]

Each body part and area of the body has its own microbial community. Different organisms live in different areas, and they are all adaptive, but the highest concentration of microbial cells in the body is in our gut.[62] The gut microbiome plays a significant rule in digestion and providing the body with essential vitamins and nutrients. People with conditions like diabetes, IBD, and Crohn's disease have a different microbiome than those without those conditions. Overweight individuals have a much less diverse microbiome than those who are lean. Even elite athletes have a very distinct type of bacteria in their gut when compared to the average person.[63]

It's no surprise that the foods we eat can have a significant impact on our microbiome and overall gut heath. Foods high in saturated fat, those sprayed with pesticides, and those that contain antibiotics that were fed to animals can alter our bacterial balance. Sometimes it's absolutely necessary to take antibiotics when we have an infection, but those antibiotics can kill the healthy bacteria in our gut. When our gut health is compromised, and we lose those healthy bacteria, more harmful microbes can create inflammation in the cell wall. This can lead to a condition called leaky gut syndrome. This is exactly what it sounds like. Food particles or organisms in the gut leak through the intestinal wall and into the bloodstream. It can be the result of any of the following conditions:

- Ulcerative colitis
- Asthma
- Crohn's disease
- Allergy
- Type 1 diabetes
- Type 2 diabetes
- Cardiovascular disease
- Non-alcoholic fatty liver disease
- Obesity
- Alcoholic liver disease
- Depression
- Irritable bowel syndrome
- Ankylosing spondylitis
- Colorectal cancer
- Chronic fatigue syndrome
- Celiac disease
- Hepatic encephalopathy
- Parkinson's disease
- Cirrhosis
- Autism spectrum disorder
- Severe acute malnutrition
- Systemic lupus erythematosus
- Necrotizing enterocolitis
- Rheumatoid arthritis

Common symptoms include:

- Gas and bloating
- Food sensitivities
- Sinus infections
- Swollen joints
- Fatigue
- Brain fog
- Skin rashes[64]

Depending on the source of the inflammation and the problem, diet and lifestyle changes are the best way to go about improving overall gut health. A healthy microbiome has a variety of bacteria, and they are always in flux. Scientists have noticed a change in the composition of the microbiome just 24 hours after an alteration in diet. Luckily, if you complete the detox, you're doing most all of this already, but when not undergoing a cleanse or detoxification program, you can take the following simple steps to help decrease the inflammation in your gut:

- Avoid refined sugars.
- Avoid milk proteins in dairy products.
- Avoid chicken protein, including eggs.
- Avoid beef and other red meats.
- Avoid soy protein.
- Avoid corn protein.
- Avoid caffeine.
- Avoid alcohol.
- Avoid NSAIDs.
- Avoid stress.[65]

While you stop doing damage to your gut, you simultaneously want to build it back up. We do that by eating foods high in fiber, like fruits, vegetables, whole grains, and legumes while avoiding fats and animal products. This is also where prebiotics and probiotics—the healthy bacteria and fungi—come into play, and the detox involves a healthy dose of both. We'll discuss these in more detail later. Glutamine and quercetin are two additional supplements that can help heal the gut. Much like the detox, these aren't meant to be permanent changes, but you do need to stop doing damage and decrease inflammation, so you can restore balance. Then you can begin reintroducing foods you normally eat back into your diet. When you do this slowly, and pay attention to how your body reacts, it better allows you to identify some of the foods you eat that might be irritating your gut.

The gut microbiome may heavily influence intestinal health, but it impacts far more than that. It's called the second brain (and the second genome) because the gut–brain axis is bidirectional in that messages and signals are sent both from the gut to the brain, and vice versa, through the vagus nerve. Your gut microbes tell your brain what to eat, and your brain tells your gut when to start the digestion process. Everything we digest has to maneuver its way through the gut. The bacteria in our gut interact with the nervous system, immune system, and endocrine system. Scientists have recently discovered that the microbiome can even influence the brain and behavior. Studies in mice have shown that the presence and absence of certain microbes can change personality. Antibiotics and probiotics have also been shown to influence the brain by influencing emotions and sensations.[66]

So many of the nutrients and supplements we're going to discuss depend on healthy microbiota in the gut to be absorbed and for us to experience the full benefit. Take pomegranate extract. This is an excellent superfood that is loaded with close to 21 polyphenols that have neuroprotective and anti-inflammatory properties that can help those with Alzheimer's among many other positive benefits.[67] However, pomegranate extract cannot cross the blood–brain barrier (which protects against unwanted substances from reaching the brain) without being bio-transformed by the gut microflora into urolithin A. So, even if you eat a healthy number of organic pomegranates, your body won't be able to absorb the polyphenols, flavonoids, and phyto-nutrients that can benefit your brain and various systems if you don't have a healthy gut. Even urolithin A has tremendous benefits, such as decreasing inflammation and improving overall cell health—just another reason to maintain a healthy gut and liver through detox. It's all connected and traces back to the gut, because everything we ingest has to be absorbed and digested, so it stands to reason that we are only as healthy as our microbiome.

Scientists are finding more links between an individual's gut microbiome and their overall level of health and aging, which is why they have been turning to the bacteria in our gut to help treat and prevent some chronic disease. If you take care of your gut, it will take care of you, and the detox is a great first step to achieving gut health. However, if you really want to know the health of your microbiome, Viome offers a great test (https://beta.viome.

com/) that can also tell you the state of your cellular health, immune system health, your biological age, and a lot of great information for a very reasonable price. They also have an app that makes for a simple user-friendly experience.

FUN FACT:

70-80 percent of our immune system is in our gut. If our body detoxes properly and our microbiome is in balance, our body is better able to fight off the common cold and the flu.[68]

ANTIOXIDANT SUPPORT

One major function of the detox is that it's loaded with antioxidants. The reason our bodies need antioxidants is because of free radicals. They are molecules with unpaired electrons that are created during digestion, exercise, exposure to toxins, by environmental factors, and when suffering from certain diseases. As a result, free radicals are unstable, and attempt to pull electrons from normal cells in the body. When free radicals are created in excess, they cause damage through oxidative stress. What's oxidative stress? Similar to how metal rusts and food goes bad, our bodies produce oxidation as we get older. Over time, this causes damage to the cells, and the cell's DNA, so that they don't replicate a healthy cell but a damaged cell. This is how our organs and or bodies age.

Antioxidants neutralize free radicals. That helps your immune system function, controls inflammation, helps alleviate some underlying health issues, and repairs damage to the cells and DNA. Our body produces what is called endogenous antioxidants, but the problem is that the body tends to make more free radicals than it does antioxidants, so we require exogenous antioxidants from food and supplements.

- ENDOGENOUS ANTIOXIDANTS: Our bodies produce the enzymes catalase, glutathione peroxidase, and superoxide dismutase. We also naturally produce the coenzymes NADH and CoQ10.
- EXOGENOUS ANTIOXIDANTS: Dietary antioxidants include vitamin A, vitamin C, vitamin E, and minerals selenium, iron, manganese, copper, zinc and sulfur compounds are vital components of antioxidant enzymes made by the body.

Exogenous antioxidants can be further broken down into subcategories including:

- CAROTENOIDS: These are pigment in plants that also serve as antioxidants. The most well-known and most important are beta-carotene, lycopene, lutein, and zeaxanthin.
- BIOFLAVONOIDS: This covers thousands of nutritional substances, and most all are found in fruits and vegetables. Like carotenoids, they also serve as plant pigments. The most well-known and important are quercetin, rutin, hesperidin, genistein, and daidzein.[69]

Most all fruits and vegetables have antioxidants, but here is a list of some of the foods with the most antioxidants:

- Coffee and tea
- Berries
- Tomatoes
- Nuts and seeds
- Dark chocolate
- Red wine
- Whole-grain bread
- Artichokes
- Pomegranates
- Curly kale[70]

You want to diversify the color of your fruits and vegetables, because different-color foods have different antioxidants. Red foods like apples, strawberries, and peppers are high in a flavonoid called anthocyanin, while orange and yellow foods, like oranges, bananas, and mangos, are a good source of vitamin C.[71] We'll go into more detail about antioxidant supplements in that chapter, but it's important to note that all of these antioxidants work together because different antioxidants protect against different types of free radicals in different cells throughout the body.

MAKING DETOX A HABIT

Even after you've completed the detox, toxins will re-enter your system, but good healthy habits can slow down that process while also making it easier for your body to secrete those toxins naturally.

I personally do two detoxes every year—a 28-day detox at the start of the new year and a 10-day detox in the summer. The new year is always a fresh start, so I do that first, more intensive detox after the holidays when we tend to slip into unhealthy eating habits. I know a couple of hardcore detox guys who do a detox during the holidays to better help them resist the temptation to indulge, but that's difficult for many to do. When the summer rolls around, there are outdoor activities, barbecues, and many opportunities to eat food I wouldn't normally eat, so I do the 10-day detox at the end of August before the kids go back to school. It's an ongoing process, but the more you can cleanse your system, the better your body (and genes) can function as intended. Twice a year is better than once a year, and once a year is better than never detoxing at all.

I've monitored hundreds of patients as they have undergone the detox program, and it's rare that someone doesn't get at least something out of it. Sometimes it's cutting out a certain food or behavior that was doing them harm; but most people change their habits. The detox is both mental and physical, so most everyone emerges thinking and feeling better.

THE EXCEPTIONS TO THE RULE

I have a patient undergoing chemotherapy, and I'm part of her team, helping her with her nutrition and supplementation while managing her side effects. She's going through cancer genomics to understand the pathway of the disease better. However, the chemo that she's undergoing actually promotes ROS, something that the detox removes. It's an interesting way to look at it, but the chemo uses the ROS to kill the cancer cells. The side effects of chemo occur because it also kills the healthy cells along with it. In a person with no health issues, the detox removes the ROS because they can destroy cellular function. My patient can't go through the detox because the antioxidants would be counterproductive and interfere with the chemo, since they eliminate ROS.

Similarly, if you're suffering from a condition like inflammatory bowel disease, I would not start with a detox because that could further inflame the gut. The detox is powerful, so we would work to heal the gut first. In those cases, I would recommend a product called Glutagenics that is designed to improve and support the damaged gastrointestinal lining. We would try that for 30 to 60 days, track any improvement, and when the gut is healthy enough to support the detox, then we would begin.

This is another reason why it's important to always consult with your physician before beginning any detox, diet, nutrition, or supplementation program. You don't know what might interfere with your body or any medication you might be taking. Even stress can complicate the process, and I would be reluctant to encourage someone to begin a detox during a stressful period of their life. It depends on you and your situation.

CHAPTER 5:

NUTRITION AND HOW TO EAT FOR YOUR GENES

Congratulations! You've completed the detox. It's now the perfect time to create sustainable change. The hard part is over. You've proven to yourself that you can eat a healthy diet that is gluten-free, dairy-free, sugar-free, and anti-inflammatory. You've probably gotten used to some of the food choices. You might even be well on your way to instinctively avoiding ingredients that you can't pronounce. That's tremendous progress. You made it over the hump and have taken a massive step in the right direction by creating some healthy habits. Why give all of that up just because the detox is over?

Let's build on that momentum and continue to make great progress. Being able to incorporate these simple nutritional strategies have helped you create positive, healthy patterns. Keep it up! Look for ways that you can make that change permanent. And this doesn't have to be a big lifestyle change. Sometimes it's the little things that can make a big difference over time. No matter your goals, here are a few tips to help you continue to progress once you've completed the detox.

1. STICK TO THE DETOX DIET

The goal of the detox is to remove toxins and inflammation from your body, but it's even better if you don't keep adding them to your system. You can't detox forever, because your body needs a break, but I encourage all of my patients to keep the detox diet going for as long as possible—specifically the eating and lifestyle habits. That doesn't mean the shakes and the antioxidants, just the recommended foods. The reason it's good to stick as closely to that diet as possible is because it's an anti-inflammatory diet, and inflammation is at the root of almost every single disease.

At the very least, try to transition into another healthy diet. If you stumbled upon a certain food you like, keep eating it. This doesn't have to be all or none. Even if you just stick to a modified detox diet five days out of the week, that can have tremendous benefits. When you keep up a healthy diet, it helps your system function better.

Before you throw in the towel, sticking to the diet is probably easier than you think. Many of us work Monday through Friday, and those days are already structured and packed, so conforming to a diet during the week is almost natural. Not only can this help you keep off any weight that you've lost, but eating healthy will help your body continue to absorb nutrients and recover. What's interesting is that since most patients look, think, and feel better after completing the detox, they want to do whatever is necessary to keep that up.

Maintaining a healthy and balanced diet of nutrient-dense foods such as fruits, vegetables, whole grains, lean protein, and healthy fats; while avoiding processed, refined, trans fats, and sugars; can help combat high cholesterol, high blood pressure, and a slew of other health ailments. Nutrition is a significant part of my practice, so I recommend that everyone eat a healthy and balanced diet.

2. DON'T BE RESTRICTIVE

Yes, you want to eat healthily, but you don't want to be miserable either. Don't starve yourself. Don't restrict yourself when it comes to food.

And don't drift too far out of your comfort zone by eating foods you don't like. Remember, the detox is not a portion-control diet. For our purposes, it doesn't matter how much you eat; what matters is that you're eating healthy foods. And even that doesn't mean you can't stray from the list every once in a while.

Give yourself the weekend, a day, or even just a meal to eat something you crave. That will help you stick to whatever healthy plan you choose to follow after the detox. Giving yourself permission to eat what you love is essential, because willpower eventually gives out. It doesn't matter who you are. If you hate what you eat, you won't stick to it, and will ultimately revert to old habits. That's not fair to yourself. That's the part that too many people forget. You have to be good to yourself. Everyone's goal is to succeed. This process isn't cheap. You're spending good money on the detox, food, and supplements, so you want to see results.

3. BUY ORGANIC FOODS

It's harder than ever to get all of the nutrients we need from our food supply, simply because the food just isn't as healthy as it was decades earlier.[72] Industrialized farming combined with waste and pollution has reduced the quality of our food supply. An apple today is far less nutritious than an apple in the 1970s.[73] Combine that with pesticides, GMOs, and other contaminants, and sometimes even our attempts to eat healthily are just another way that we're putting toxins in our body. Not only could the strawberries you're buying contain various toxins, but so could the plastic container and that packet on the bottom of the container used to keep the product fresh. That's why I always recommend that my patients buy organic foods whenever possible. Yes, I know organic food is more expensive, but where you get your food is just as important as where it comes from, how far it had to travel, and where it was stored. When I first started my practice, this type of information was limited, but as our society becomes more health-conscious, it is more readily available. That better allows us to make sure that we can purchase the best-quality food possible if we desire. Paying just a little bit more attention to the source of your food can have a positive impact on your body, your health, and your genes.

4. *LOOK FOR HEALTHIER ALTERNATIVES*

Lauren was a patient who loved licorice. She not only ate it every single day, but she knew everything there was to know about licorice. It was fascinating to listen to her talk about it, but the FDA has warned that eating high amounts of licorice could lead to arrhythmia, high blood pressure, and other heart issues.[74]

We tested Lauren's DNA, she went through the detox, and we put her on a nutrition and supplement plan, but she still couldn't cut out her favorite snack. Eventually, we found a pure source of licorice that was much less harmful to her, and she made the switch. That proved to be the best of both worlds.

We all have weaknesses when it comes to food. Be honest with yourself about what yours are, because if the food you love is unhealthy, you might be able to find something similar that is just as satisfying yet much better for your body.

5. *PAY ATTENTION TO HOW YOUR FOOD IS PREPARED*

Steaming, grilling, or deep frying—if given a choice, what method do you typically choose? How about stir frying, baking, sautéing, poaching, roasting, steaming, broiling, and grilling? You have a lot of choices when it comes to how you prepare your food, but yes, some methods are better than others. Here is a quick guide:

- STEAMING: This is one of the most efficient methods of preserving nutrient content. It also works relatively quickly. If given the choice, steam your food.
- BOILING: This can strip foods, especially vegetables, of their nutrient content. The greater amount of water being used leads to greater nutrient loss.
- FRYING: What you gain in taste and efficiency when frying, you lose in nutrients. You might add free radicals, and possibly carcinogens, to the food during the process.

- STIR-FRYING: Better than deep frying, stir-frying is still a form of frying, which means nutrients can be lost and fats chemically altered.
- MICROWAVING: When it comes to vegetables, microwaving is better than boiling, but still not as good as steaming for retaining nutrients.
- ROASTING: Beef, chicken, and fish can be safely roasted while retraining nutrients, but when burned, free radicals and carcinogens are created. The longer the food is roasted, and the higher the temperature, the greater the nutrient loss.
- BARBECUING: People love to barbecue in the summer, but when the fat from meat drips onto the flame of the grill, carcinogens can form in the smoke and be absorbed into the meat.[75]
- RAW FOOD: Aside from meat products that need to be cooked, eating raw food is the healthiest option and the best way to benefit from all the nutrients of fruits, vegetables, nuts, grains, and seeds.[76]

This doesn't mean that you can never eat fried foods. You just want to be careful about how you prepare them. When my kids want French fries, we buy potatoes from the store, cut them up at home, and fry them in the deep fryer using grape seed oil. We only use that oil once, so it's much healthier than if we were to cook more food in the same oil. It's the same thing with barbecuing in that it all comes down to how you do it. Try choosing leaner meats, remove any skin or excess fat, and don't cook your meat directly over the flame.

FUN FACT:

Sugary drinks are the most fattening product in the modern diet, and our brain doesn't compensate for the calories by eating less food. If anything, we tend to eat more overall.[77]

DR. M'S MODIFIED MEDITERRANEAN DIET

It's important to remember that the main purpose of food is to fuel our bodies. It does so primarily through three macronutrients:

- Carbohydrates: This is the main energy source for the body and brain. These are grains, starches, fruits, and vegetables. During digestion, they are broken down into glucose, which provides energy for your muscles.

- Fats: These provide the structural foundation for your cells and hormones. You can get healthy fats from oil, butter, cream, olives, avocados, and other foods. Without enough fat, your brain, skin, hair, bones, reproductive system, immune system, energy levels, and ability for your blood to clot can all be compromised.

- Proteins: These are the building blocks that repair and build muscle, including the muscles that operate your organs. You get healthy protein from dairy foods, nuts, and animal products.

These all provide different combinations of vitamins and minerals that influence our metabolism, health, and overall function; but they also work together. So the key is to find the right balance. But what is that balance, and what foods should you eat?

It would be ideal for everyone to be on a vegetarian or vegan diet, but that just isn't practical. Some people have no problem going vegan, but many struggle because it's too restrictive. You want to make changes that you can sustain, so it doesn't do you any good to be a strict vegan for two months and then resort back to old ways. That's why I personally believe the Mediterranean diet is the most optimal out of all the popular diets. The three macronutrients (carbohydrates, protein, and fat) are well balanced, and it's loaded with antioxidants and minerals that can help keep cholesterol and blood sugar levels in a healthy range. Following this diet involves avoiding sugar, starchy foods, trans fats, and red meat.

Studies in Spain found that the Mediterranean diet led to beneficial changes in metabolic syndrome, blood pressure, lipid profiles, inflammation, oxidative stress, and carotid atherosclerosis. From a genetic standpoint, recent research determined that the Mediterranean diet could modulate the expression of genes linked to inflammation and atherosclerosis. The diet may also reduce the risk of cardiovascular disease by reducing homocysteine concentrations in nearly 60 percent of the population while also influencing methylation.[78]

When it comes to eating for your genes, I've put my own spin on the Mediterranean diet. I've added more gamey, lean meats and wild-caught fish instead of beef and pork. That's easier for people to digest, and it's a healthier alternative for those with cardiovascular disease, high cholesterol, autoimmune diseases, and pro-inflammatory conditions.

This modified Mediterranean diet is what I recommend to most of my patients, especially if they have a sensitivity to carbohydrates or saturated fats. I've seen patients experience better results with this diet when it comes to improving chronic conditions including heart disease, diabetes, and cancer.

Much like the detox diet, this is not about portion control, though some of my patients want everything to be measured and even buy food scales. Other patients want a generalized idea of what they have to do, and they can be specific with how they execute it. One approach is not better than the other, but everyone is different, so you have to find what works best for you. What's most important is that you stick to the foods on the list. It's about finding the right balance of macronutrients—fats, proteins, carbohydrates, and minerals—and knowing where to get them and how to cook them. That, to me, is more important than portion control. It's about improving your relationship with food.

THE BASIC RULES

- Gluten-free. Even avoid foods that mimic gluten, like millet, oats, and yeast.
- Casein-free.
- Limit intake of excitotoxins (a class of chemicals or amino acids that overstimulate the nervous system, such as MSG and

aspartame) and xenobiotics (substances that are foreign to the body, such as toxins like lead or mercury).

- Limit exposure to mercury and aluminum.
- Limit intake of saponins like quinoa and nightshades like tomato, potato, eggplant, bell pepper, and chili peppers. Nightshades contain alkaloids that, in extremely high doses, can increase inflammation and potentially be poisonous. [79]
- Limit intake of lectins because they contain phytohaemagglutinin, which can cause red blood cells to clump and lead to gas, bloating, nausea, vomiting, upset stomach, and diarrhea. Boiling, stewing, or soaking lectins in water can inactivate them.[80]
- Avoid GMOs. There are currently eight genetically engineered crops on the U.S. market: corn, soybean, cotton, canola, alfalfa, sugar beets, papaya, and squash. [81]
- Avoid ALL sugars. You can substitute Stevia or Monk Fruit when applicable.
- Limit salt intake, but when you do use salt, you want to make sure that it contains iodine.

HERE'S WHAT YOU CAN EAT

- FRUITS: All berries, apples, apricots, avocado, bananas, cantaloupe, cherries, coconut, fig, guava, honeydew, kiwi, kumquat, lemon, lime, loquat, lychee, mango, nectarines, olive, orange, papaya, passionfruit, peach, pear, persimmon, pineapple, plum, pomegranate, pomelo, quince, star fruit, and watermelon.
- VEGETABLES: artichoke (globe/heart/Jerusalem), arugula, asparagus, avocado, beets, bok choy, broccoli, Brussels sprouts, cabbage, carrots, cauliflower, chives, celery, collard greens, cucumbers, fennel, garlic, jicama, kale, leeks, mushrooms, mustard greens, onions, parsnips, pumpkin, radishes, rhubarb, rutabaga, sea veggies, shallots, spinach, squash, yams, Swiss chard, watercress, and zucchini.
- LAND: bison/ buffalo, boar, chicken (only organic), duck, elk, emu, goose, lamb, ostrich, pheasant, quail, veal, venison, and yak.

▷ Try to get your meats from markets like Harmony Farms, Whole Foods, Bristol Farms, or trusted farmer's markets.

- SEA: Anchovies, branzino, butterfish, calamari, halibut, herring, mackerel (North Atlantic/chub), mullet, pollock, salmon, sardine, sole, and tilapia.

- NUTS: Almonds, Brazil nuts, cashews, chia seeds, flaxseeds, pistachios, and walnuts.

- FERMENTED FOODS: Coconut kefir, naturally fermented pickles, kimchi, kombucha, olives, and sauerkraut.

- SPICES AND CONDIMENTS: Apple cider vinegar, basil, bay leaf, black pepper, peppercorns, chives, coriander, cumin, dandelion, dill, Fennel seed, garlic, ginger, oregano, parsley, rosemary, tarragon, thyme, and turmeric.

  ▷ Look for organic, non-irradiated, non-GMO brands. My favorite is Frontier Co-op.

- BONE BROTH: Only organic. Homemade preferred.

COOKING OILS AND DRESSING OILS

Oils and fats can have a significant impact on your overall cardiovascular health, so when deciding what oils to use for dressing and cooking, you want to make sure that you're making the healthiest possible choice. There are three categories of fatty acids. Put simply, here is how it breaks down:

- Saturated Fats and Oils: Butter fat, animal fat, coconut oil, palm oil, and cocoa butter.

  ▷ These raise bad cholesterol (LDL) and blood pressure.

- Monosaturated Oils: Olive oil, canola oil, high oleic safflower oil, high oleic sunflower oil, and avocado oil.

  ▷ These raise good cholesterol (HDL), lower bad cholesterol (LDL), and can lower blood pressure.

- Polysaturated Oils: Corn oil, safflower oil, sunflower oil, peanut oil, cottonseed oil, canola oil (high in both polysaturated and monosaturated oil), soybean oil, fish oil, flaxseed oil, walnut oil, primrose oil, sesame oil, grapeseed oil, and borage oil.

> ▷ Polysaturated oils can further be broken down into two main categories, though there is some overlap.

- Omega-3 Oils: Fish oil, canola oil, flaxseed oil, walnut oil, and soybean oil.
  - These can raise good cholesterol (HDL), while causing bad cholesterol (LDL) to go up or down. They can also lower blood pressure and risk of blood clotting. This makes them a good replacement for saturated fats like fatty meat, butter, eggs, cheese, and whole milk.
- Omega-6 Oils: Corn oil, safflower oil, and sunflower oil.
  - When you balance your Omega-6 and Omega-3 oils, you have a much lower risk of inflammatory diseases.[82] You want to favor Omega-3 (anti-inflammatory) over Omega-6 (pro-inflammatory). An increased use of processed vegetable oils has caused the average American to have a much higher level of Omega-6s, but it's best to have a low, balanced amount of each. I use the Nutr Eval Test from Genova Diagnostics, and it recommends a range between 3.4 and 10.7.

Given their various properties, some of these oils are better for cooking and some are better for dressing. One reason is because the properties of certain oils can change when heated. It often comes down to the smoking point, which is the temperature oil can be heated to before it smokes and begins to decompose.

At our house, we use grapeseed oil for cooking oil and olive oil for dressing oil. The smoking point of grapeseed oil is about 420 degrees Fahrenheit, and the smoking point of olive oil is between 374 degrees and 405 degrees Fahrenheit. When olive oil starts to smoke, it becomes unstable and changes chemically from an unsaturated fat to trans fat, which makes it potentially harmful. It's saturated fat and trans-fatty acids that, in combination with inflammation, can clog arteries and lead to heart disease and cardiovascular disease. Rancid and oxidized oil can also create free radicals, which can attack and damage our DNA. In their book *The Food Doctor*, Vicki Edgson and Ian Marber compare DNA replication to a photocopier, because if the original document is damaged or has blemishes, then the copies will as well.[83] It's the same with our DNA, so we want to avoid damaging our DNA whenever possible.

The heating point of grapeseed oil, a polyunsaturated fat, is much higher and doesn't undergo the same chemical change, so I highly recommend using grapeseed oil as a cooking oil instead of olive oil. However, olive oil works exceptionally well as a dressing oil. It can also decrease the risk of blood clots because it has squalene, which has anticlotting properties and can lower cholesterol. The body can break down unsaturated fats and use them as energy. But since heat can change its composition, you want to store them in dark glass bottles, so the oil doesn't get oxidized by the sun or the heat because the composition would change, and it could become harmful, just as it would when you heat it up. But these aren't your only options. Here are some others:

- COOKING OILS: Ghee/clarified butter, coconut oil, grapeseed oil, safflower oil, peanut oil and refined almond, avocado, and cottonseed oils.
- DRESSING OILS: Olive oil, avocado oil, high-oleic unrefined organic sunflower oil.

FUN FACT:

Eating fast causes a stress response leading to a slower metabolism, reduced calorie-burning capacity, reduced vitamin and mineral absorption, and reduced muscle-building. So, slow down when you eat![84]

What you eat is important, but you also want to consider what you eat that food with because certain foods pair well with other foods. Think of it this way: When you sit down for a meal, the food blends together and ends up all in the same place. However, different enzymes break down different foods during digestion, but since all the different foods are combined together, the enzymes don't always attach to the right molecules. This can lead to gas, bloating, diarrhea, and a host of intestinal issues. Over an extended period of time, it can even lead to chronic disease. That's why proper food synergy is essential so the digestive system can function properly and help you achieve optimal health

Typically speaking, carbohydrates are good to mix with fats, while proteins are not. However, proteins, fats, and carbohydrates are all good to mix with non-starchy green vegetables. Here is a quick guide of specific foods that do mix well together:

- Eat protein with vegetables.
- Eat fruits with fruits and citrus with citrus.
- Oil and starches.
- Avocado (considered a protein) and low-level starches and acid fruits.
- Tomatoes and low-starchy vegetables, nuts, and avocado.
- Celery and lettuce with all vegetables (except melon).
- Soaked nuts (protein) and citrus.
- Starchy foods with vegetables.
- Nuts and seeds (protein) with leafy greens.
- Papaya goes with all foods.

Foods you want to avoid mixing:

- Avoid mixing protein with starches.
- Avoid mixing melon with other foods.
- Avoid acidic fruits (grapefruit, apples, oranges, cherries) with other foods.
- Avoid sweet fruits (bananas, grapes) with other foods.

- Avoid multiple types of starches with one meal.[85]

DNA-RECOMMENDED MODIFICATIONS

When it comes to health and nutrition, there are many different variables to consider, which is why you must always consult with your physician. And before you make any post-detox diet plans, you should also take another look at your genome, because that can further influence what you eat. I keep saying that there's no one-size-fits-all solution, which still applies to diets and nutrition, but genetic predispositions can change how your body processes certain nutrients, making some diets more optimal than others. Based on your genetic profile, you might learn that your body might be better suited for and respond better to one of the following four diet plans.

1. LOW-CARB DIET

If your DNA test reveals an average genetic likelihood for elevated blood sugar levels, or if you just want to monitor your insulin and blood sugar while avoiding metabolic syndrome, a low-carb diet might be beneficial. This means avoiding starchy carbs like white bread and potatoes in favor of vegetables, healthy fats, and lean protein. Atkins and Keto are two popular versions of a low-carb diet, but your daily carb intake depends on your goals.

- 100 to 150 grams is intended for weight maintenance or frequent high-intensity exercise.
- 50 to 100 grams is intended for slow and steady weight loss.
- Under 50 grams is intended for fast weight loss.[86]

The opposite is true as well, and your genes might be the reason why you tried the Atkins diet, Keto, or any other popular diet and didn't see the results you desired, despite following the program perfectly. Many genes are involved in energy metabolism, including variants of the APOE gene, which determines if more or fewer carbohydrates are suitable for your cholesterol levels. For example, APOE4 carriers are better suited for high-carbohydrate, low-fat diets, while APOE2 carriers are better suited for low-carbohydrate, high-fat diets.[87]

2. LOW-FAT DIET

There are hundreds of genes linked to various aspects of weight gain, appetite, our ability to burn calories, our body composition, glucose absorption, and metabolism. Some of the most significant are:

- FTO. This protein associated with fat mass and obesity is found on chromosome 16, and those with this gene have a 30 percent higher chance of being overweight.
- MC4R. This gene impacts metabolism and controls how much energy we use from food and our feelings of hunger. A variant of this gene often results in people being overweight.
- ANKYRIN-B. A variant of this gene causes fat cells to absorb glucose at an accelerated rate, which increases the size of the cell and can lead to obesity.
- PANX1. This gene regulates the accumulation of fat and is connected with a higher rate of obesity.
- IRX3. Those with this gene may experience difficulty losing weight. Studies showed that those with deficient expressions of this gene experienced a 30 percent loss in weight.[88]

A genetic predisposition to high cholesterol may be combated with a simple low-fat diet. Experts recommend that on a 2,000-calories-per-day diet, adults get between 20 and 25 percent of their daily calories from fat. That translates to about 44 to 77 grams of fat a day.[89] Fifty-five to 60 percent of calories would derive from carbohydrates and 20 percent from protein.

With this diet, the type of fat you eat is important, and you want to eliminate saturated and trans fats in favor of healthier unsaturated fats. Here's a quick breakdown:

- *Unsaturated Fats*: Heart-healthy fats that can be divided into monounsaturated fats like avocado, olives, nuts, and nut butters, and polyunsaturated fats like omega 3s (walnuts, flaxseeds, and fish), and omega 6s (vegetable oils and seeds).
- *Saturated fats:* These are non-essential fats like animal fats (red meat, poultry skin, dairy products, eggs, cream, butter, and lard),

tropical oils (coconut products), and also more hidden saturated fats (milk powders, coffee creamers, and ice cream). These should be kept to a minimum.

- *Trans Fats:* These are non-essential fats like margarine, baked goods, pastries, chips, and fried foods that you should limit if not remove altogether.

As often is the case, nature and nurture are each at play. For example, studies showed that the APOA2 gene could impact a person's weight and BMI if they had diets high in saturated fats, but those with the gene who didn't eat a diet high in saturated fat didn't experience weight gain.[90] It just goes to show that by eating a healthy diet while exercising regularly and living an overall healthy lifestyle, you can avoid so many preventable conditions that you might not even know you're predisposed to.

3. LACTOSE-FREE DIET

Lactose intolerance can lead to a host of gastrointestinal symptoms. The first step is avoiding the sugar found in milk and replacing it with alternatives like almond milk or oat milk. Other foods to avoid are cheese, butter, yogurt, ice cream, frozen yogurt, buttermilk, sour cream, and whipped cream. Some prepared foods also contain dairy products, so it's important to check labels to find which meals, baked goods, and candies might contain lactose.

It's recommended that you attempt to go 30 days without eating any dairy to see if symptoms improve; but whether or not the condition improves depends on the cause. Many factors can influence lactose intolerance, both genetic and non-genetic. For example, a mutation in the LCT gene, which contains instructions for making the enzyme lactase, leads to low lactose levels in the gut and creates complications when digesting dairy products.[91] Many genomic companies, include 23andMe, AxGen, and Prometheus, test for the LCT gene mutation.

4. GLUTEN-FREE DIET

Gluten is the protein found in grains including wheat, spelt, barley (malt), rye, oats, and kamut. It's primarily made of two proteins: prolamins and glutenins. It's sometimes used in dough and some sauces. It can also be found in medicine, toothpaste, and cosmetics. There is a wide range of gluten-free products that can be beneficial, particularly if you're suffering from gluten sensitivity or gluten intolerance. However, many people have a fundamental misunderstanding of the difference between the two.

Sensitivities and allergies are often confused, but they are very different, and it comes down to your body's reaction. An allergy is caused by the immune system, while a sensitivity can be traced to the digestive system. Allergies are caused by IgE antibodies, and can lead to tongue swelling, itching, rash, rapid heartbeat, nausea, vomiting, dizziness, shortness of breath, difficulty breathing and even some life-threatening symptoms. When it comes to food sensitivities, they are IgG-mediated, and there are multiple theories of sources, but the most common is a dysfunctional gut lining stemming from weakened tight junctions that keep the cells of the GI tract locked together. When this lining is weakened, it can lead to leaky gut and can cause an immune response. Dietary and lifestyle factors such as alcohol, stress, NSAIDs, prolonged strenuous exercise, and Western-type diets high in red meat, animal fat, and sugar can all contribute to various food sensitivities, including gluten sensitivity.

IgE-Mediated Allergies (Foods, molds, inhalants)	IgG-Mediated Sensitivities (Foods, spices, vegetarian foods)
*Immediate onset (minutes to hours)	*Delayed onset (hours to days)
*Circulation half-life of 1 to 2 days	*Temporary sensitivities
*Permanent allergies	*Activates complement System
*Stimulates histamine release	*Does not stimulate histamine release
*Symptoms: hives, stuffy or itchy nose, sneezing, itchy, teary eyes, vomiting, stomach cramps, diarrhea, angioedema or swelling, shortness of breath or wheezing, anaphylaxis.	*Gastrointestinal symptoms, headache, other vague symptoms.[92]

Three main types of gluten intolerances include:

1. Wheat Allergy: This is an allergic response by the body that can lead to rashes, asthma, and anaphylactic shock, but does not destroy body tissue.

2. Celiac Disease: This is an autoimmune disease that requires a strict avoidance of gluten. It's a genetic condition that can lead to damage of the small intestine. Symptoms include weight loss, watery stools, stomach pain, vomiting, fatigue, bloating, and distension.[93] Prolamins (a group of plant storage proteins) are directly connected to Celiac disease and make up a significant protein percentage of the following grains:

- Wheat – 69%
- Rye – 30-50%
- Oats – 12-16%
- Barley – 46-52%
- Millet – 40%
- Corn – 55%
- Rice – 5%
- Sorghum – 54%
- Teff – 11%

3. Non-Celiac Gluten Sensitivity (NCGS): This is the inability to tolerate gluten, and even though it's much less severe than Celiac disease, the symptoms are similar and include bloating, gas, abdominal pain, diarrhea, and constipation. However, the intestinal damage is not as significant as Celiac disease, but they often include symptoms that exist outside of the gut, such as headache, brain fog, nausea, joint pain, depression, anemia, and numbness in the limbs and extremities. These symptoms can appear hours and days after ingesting gluten.[94] Everyone is different, and there is no one-size-fits-all guideline for how much gluten you can consume before falling ill. It's not a case of how much gluten you want to include in your diet as it is how little gluten it will take to negatively impact you.

If you feel this is an issue, the first step is getting tested for Celiac disease and a wheat allergy. If both of those tests are negative, you can also take a food intolerance test—Genova Diagnostics has a great test. However, your DNA might hold some clues, and the gold standard for identifying NCGS is genomic testing. It is important to note that roughly 3 million people, or 1 percent of the population, actually have Celiac disease.[95] However, it's estimated that between 35 and 40 percent of the population have the celiac disease genes: HLA DQ2 or HLA DQ8, while some believe that those with HLA DQ1 and HLA DQ3 are predisposed to having gluten sensitivity.[96] Other genes associated with gluten sensitivity include FLG, CTNNA3, and RBFOX1.[97] The Glutenomics website that I created (www.glutenomics.com) has the most advanced Genetic test for gluten sensitivities, Celiac Disease and for determining predictive risk for developing Celiac Disease in the world. Glutenomics is the only company that tests all the major HLA- DQ gene versions, along with thousands more. We have partnered with AxGen out of need for more DNA and genomics precision medicine for predisposition to gluten sensitivities and allergens.

Before beginning any treatment, you want to notify your primary care physician and follow their specific instructions. Those instructions most often involve eliminating the culprit—gluten. You will have to do this permanently for Celiac disease, and if you have a wheat allergy, you need to permanently eliminate wheat from your diet. For NCGS, you want to temporarily eliminate gluten to see if your symptoms improve. The elimination diet is a good way to identify any potential cross-reactivity food that may also cause a reaction. In my experience, all three conditions are often an indication of localized tissue damage and other systematic concerns. That's why I highly recommend conventional lab testing, and functional lab testing to address those systemic issues. In my own practice, I use the following three tests from Cyrex Labs.[98]

- Array #5: Multiple Autoimmune Reactivity Screen.
- Array #3x: Wheat/Gluten Proteome Reactivity.
- Array #10: Multiple Food Immune Reactivity Screen.

FUN FACT:

The truth is that organic sugar is still sugar, and gluten-free junk food is still junk food.[99]

COMBATTING METABOLIC SYNDROME

Believe it or not, it's your nutritional choices and not your genetics that can ultimately determine your overall health later in life and whether or not you develop certain diseases that you are genetically predisposed to.

James, a 40-year-old client of mine, went to have bloodwork done when he wasn't feeling well and learned that he was pre-diabetic. This was a concern because his father had diabetes, developed heart disease, and ended up on dialysis. According to the American Diabetes Association, diabetes results in chronic inflammation, so it can lead to serious complications such as nerve damage, eye conditions (which may lead to blindness), skin conditions, cardiovascular diseases, high blood pressure, foot complications (which may lead to amputations), kidney disease, and stroke.[100] I see this a lot, and it's called metabolic syndrome—a cluster of conditions including high-blood pressure, high blood sugar, excess body fat, and high cholesterol levels that increase the risk of heart disease, stroke, and diabetes.

To avoid this, we immediately conducted a genomic analysis and tested 24 genes directly related to heart disease and diabetes to give us the rough percentage that he would have of developing those diseases. He had 13 genes linked to type 2 diabetes, and that made sense because that's what his father had, and since his mom didn't have diabetes, he most likely inherited these genes from his father.

The advantage with this client is that he was only 40, so he had a choice. He could continue eating a diet that is not compatible with his genome that will most likely lead to him developing conditions similar to his father, or he could take control of his diet and make healthy changes that can improve the quality of his life.

In 20 or 30 years, we might reach a point where the CRISPR/Cas9 technology will allow us to remove these harmful genes. Scientists have already been able to use CRISPR to remove a gene that lowers blood cholesterol levels in mice.[101] Until this technology is safe and ethical to use on humans, nutrigenomics is the best weapon you have to protect yourself against developing certain conditions. Time will tell what this client will choose to do, but now that he's aware of his situation, he has the opportunity to prevent himself from suffering the same fate as his father.

FUN FACT:

The obesity rate in adults in the United States stood at 42.4% in the year 2020, which had increased from 26% in 2008. The obesity rate in the European region was above 51.6% in 2014 and is continuously rising.[102]

EATING FOR YOUR NUCLEOTIDES

When I was in chiropractic school, they taught us how the problem you're experiencing is only the tip of the iceberg, and most of what's really going on occurs underneath the surface. So, if you have a headache, you have to find the cause to really treat the headache. Is it a migraine, tension headache, or a tumor? It's the same with any disease. What's the source? When you trace it all the way through the body, you get down to proteins, cells, and eventually DNA.

DNA is the basis of our existence, and it's made up of three parts: Sugar, phosphate, and nucleic acid or base pairs: adenine (A), thymine (T), cytosine (C), and guanine (G).

This is your instruction manual for life. It's your blueprint for what makes you YOU, and it impacts the way you think, act, feel, and if you get a particular disease. So, if you have a malfunction at a cellular level, it can manifest through certain conditions that show up during physical exams, blood work, functional medicine tests, and during other routine health checkups. There are ways to strengthen our DNA, specifically the nucleotides, through nutrition and supplementation. In essence, it's how we safeguard our existence. One way to start is by eating specific foods:

- ORGAN MEATS: Beef liver, beef kidney, beef heart, beef brain, pork liver, chicken liver, chicken heart.
- FRESH SEAFOOD: Anchovies, clams, mackerel, salmon, sardines, squid.
- DRIED LEGUMES: Garbanzo beans, split peas, lentils, blackeye peas, pinto beans.

A French diet is rich in these foods, and I've personally dubbed eating for your nucleotides "the New French Paradox."

The gut and the liver are the two main organs involved in the production of nucleotides. When you take in food from the outside, it has to go through the gut and the liver, so you want to maintain the integrity of those organs and keep them as healthy as possible. This connects back to having a healthy microbiome and how that can aid in DNA synthesis.

If your nucleotides remain healthy, that can help with the aging process. The body needs to create new cells every minute because it must create new cells as fast as old cells die. It relies on DNA and RNA to do this, and that requires a significant number of nucleotides. Think of it this way—normal DNA contains three billion nucleotide pairs.[103] Why not feed them the food necessary to keep them healthy?

QUALITY COFFEE AND WHERE TO GET IT

An AP poll has found that America is a nation in a hurry.[104] This is especially true in the morning. A lot of people get in the habit of taking their supplements with their morning coffee. Now, as great as coffee is in many ways, it does block the absorption of B vitamins.[105] This can especially be a problem if you have a mutation that leaves you deficient in B vitamins and take supplements with your coffee to make up for that deficiency. I recommend that people get out of the habit of taking supplements with their coffee and wait a few hours after taking vitamins to have their morning coffee, so you can better absorb any B vitamins.

It's not just the coffee itself but how it's processed that is also a problem. Because of how the caffeine is harvested, extracted from the beans, dried, cleaned, washed, hauled, and sorted, there might be chemicals that promote cancer in some more popular coffee products. The way the beans are mechanically harvested, and any additional preservatives, can add additional chemicals. Three brands of coffee are considered by connoisseurs to be the best quality:

- Mavis Bank—Jamaican Blue Mountain Coffee
- Kona Coffee—Hawaii
- Papua New Guinea—Sigri Estate A

These are definitely not the average everyday coffees because they are more expensive than the typical brands, but they contain the purest form of caffeine. The beans are handpicked and dried through much more natural methods, so they aren't massively produced. And since there aren't any additional chemicals or preservatives, they have a much shorter expiration date.

ALCOHOL, MARIJUANA, AND DRUGS

One of the genes I look at for my patients are CB1 and AKT1, which play a role in the likelihood of developing marijuana-induced paranoia and even psychosis in mega-doses.[106] Some of my patients who have these genes have in fact reported that when they smoked marijuana, they didn't find it enjoyable, and experienced feelings of paranoia. It created a negative effect and didn't sit well with them. The reason is because these genes play a role in how the body processes marijuana, and if you have these genes, the higher the THC content in a marijuana product, the more dangerous it becomes.

In those cases, it's best to avoid synthetic and mega doses of THC in favor of products that contain more CBD and less THC.

Genetics also plays a role in how your body processes alcohol, which can lead to some with certain genes and enzymes (ADH1B, ADH1C, and ALDH2) to have a greater risk of alcoholism. This can also lead to a number of conditions, such as liver cirrhosis, stomach cancer, and even Alzheimer's disease. This is also true of certain ethnic groups as well. For example, studies have found that there is a genetic component for substance abuse in certain Native American tribes.[107] There are symptoms that might indicate you have a certain mutation, such as facial flushing or redness of the face after consuming alcohol. Before you indulge in recreational substances, you might want to look at your genes, and see if you might have an enzyme or mutation that prevents your body from properly processing that substance.

When it comes to any prescription medications, if you ever have any questions about how the drugs you take interact with your body and genome, the go-to site is https://www.pharmgkb.org/. PharmaGKB is a great site that can be extremely helpful because it has so much information. I had a patient who learned he was a slow metabolizer of acetaminophen, which is the most common over-the-counter pain-relieving drug, and what's used in Tylenol. Since this accumulates in his body, he requires a lower dosage. Until you check, you have no idea how your body might be processing some of the prescriptions you take every single day.

FUN FACT:

These days, food engineers have found ways to make food so rewarding that your brain gets flooded with dopamine. Many studies examining this phenomenon have found similarities between processed junk foods and commonly abused drugs.[108]

DNA NUTRITION APPS

If following nutritional guidelines feels overwhelming, and you know that it will be difficult for you to stay on track, consider using an app. Some people find these helpful, and others don't. It all depends on personal preference, but many DNA nutrition apps on the market do most of the same things we've discussed. Much like the genomic DNA tests, different companies specialize in different areas, so you have to find the one that best fits your needs. Technology is increasing rapidly, but here are a few of the products on the market as of this book's writing.

- DNA DIET. Personalized weight loss tailored to your genes that shows you how variations in your DNA cause you to react to certain foods.
- HEALTHY NUTRITION. Use your genetics to determine your body's unique responses to certain foods, as well as guidance when it comes to various nutrients and foods.
- NUTRITION HERITAGE REPORT. Learn where your nutrition genes came from and receive guidance on helping choose foods optimal for your genetics.
- NUTRITION REPORT. This is a more comprehensive overview of how your DNA influences your body's response to your diet.
- NOURISH. Customized diet advice on what to eat based on 26 traits, 50 genes, and 68 SNPs.
- LEAN AND FIT. Optimized fitness and daily wellness plans based on your genetics. Learn your optimal combination of exercise, nutrition, psychology, and skincare to achieve your goals.
- EMPOWER. A custom evaluation and health enrichment plan of your nutrition, exercise, and sleep based on 20 traits, 37 genes, and 53 SNPs.

CHAPTER 6:

THE IMPORTANCE OF QUALITY SUPPLEMENTATION

As we get older, certain parts of the body, and the way they function, decline. It's just a fact of life. Men lose testosterone with age, and women lose estrogen and progesterone. Both men and women can suffer general hormone imbalances, and changes to their overall gut health because as we age, so does the microbiome. Dysbiosis is a shift in the microbiome that can lead to inflammation. Meanwhile, healthy microbes are replaced with those that can cause illness.[109] The thyroid may become nodular with age, and that can slow down your metabolism. Weight gain, muscle loss, memory loss, fertility issues, mood swings, decreased libido, hair loss, and sleeping issues are all common as we age.

So it should be no surprise that you can't expect to eat the same foods when you're in your 40s and 50s as you did when you were in your 20s and expect to maintain the same weight and overall level of health. You have to change your diet, but sometimes diet alone isn't enough. Food is an excellent source of vitamins, minerals, and nutrients, but when it comes to getting your proper daily allowances, you have to eat so much of certain foods that it's not practical to even try. Couple this with the decrease of digestive juices and the GI motility as we age, digestion and the absorption of key nutrients decreases. In my experience, this becomes a vicious cycle that creates systemic inflammation and the overall feeling of being unwell. This is where supplementation comes in, but what supplements should you take?

People mean well, and they want to get better—some are willing to try everything. They might hear about certain products from friends, on television, or even from their own research on the internet (Dr. Google). They hear what worked for someone else and then read about the latest trend and how helpful it can be. Pretty soon, they are taking a ton of supplements just to take them without really understanding how or if what they're taking will have any impact.

Genomics can help you cut through the noise. Once you have your DNA raw data, it allows you to effectively take supplements for a purpose. When I received my genetic test results a few years ago, I learned that I had inherited several genes for cardiovascular disease and diabetes from my dad, which meant that I was predisposed to those diseases. I was almost 50 and didn't have any issues, but I immediately took the proper preventative methods by ordering the appropriate supplements. That's specialized medicine at its finest. Think of an iceberg and how the symptoms we experience are only the tip, above the water. With genomics, we can go to the source, that section of the iceberg underneath the water that isn't visible on the surface. That's how you can protect yourself from certain health conditions before they arise.

FUN FACT:

The word "vitamine" was first coined by Polish biochemist Casimir Funk in 1920, and derives from the Latin word "vita," meaning life, and "amine," since scientists first believed they contained amino acids.[110]

YOU GET WHAT YOU PAY FOR

I feel for my patients. I know they are coming to me for help. Many have gone everywhere else, and nothing has worked, so they feel like they have gotten the short end of the stick. I want to restore their faith by giving them a quality product that will get the results. But when it comes to choosing supplements, the rule of thumb is that you get what you pay for. That doesn't mean expensive is always better, but the source of the supplements you're taking is important because supplements aren't regulated by the FDA.[111] That means the products differ drastically in terms of absorption, quality, and potency. Today, the supplements you can purchase in the United States can be broken up into three categories.

1. DIRECT TO CONSUMER

These are the supplements you see on the shelf of any grocery store or health food store. These are the supplements that are mass-produced for the general public. If you are already taking supplements, they are most likely from this first category.

2. THROUGH A PROVIDER

Several companies only provide supplements to qualified licensed practitioners, and these are primarily the supplements I recommend for my patients. In general, supplements don't require a prescription, but this is the closest you get to prescription and pharmaceutical quality.

3. BASED ON YOUR GENOME

This option is becoming more popular, as there are companies like Pure Encapsulation, Holistic Health, and Regener8[112] that send a test kit to your home, and you return a swab with your DNA. They then customize a supplement plan based on your genome. They are the first company I've seen who has provided this service, but I'm sure more will soon follow.

WHAT'S THE DIFFERENCE?

Sure, you can go down to the nearest health food store and buy a very affordable bottle of glucosamine sulfate that is much less expensive than the glucosamine sulfate made by the companies that only supply licensed practitioners. The name on the label might be the same, but the product can be very different. How so?

Only about three percent of the supplements on the market are professional grade, or Practitioner grade and the main difference is ingredient quality, concentration and purity. Practitioner grade supplements contain the purest form of the nutrient while ensuring maximum absorption. Even though no product can ever be 100 percent pure, these supplements don't contain any binders, fillers, or unknown substances.

It all starts with the raw material, because the better the raw material, the purer the supplement. Take a supplement like chondroitin, which helps aid in osteoarthritis. Like glucosamine, it is a normal part of cartilage that can be produced from natural sources (like shark or bovine cartilage), or it can also be produced in the lab. It's the same product, but you wouldn't get the same quality nutrients in a supplement produced in a lab as you would a supplement that used natural sources. Since natural sources are more difficult to extract, that can be the difference between a supplement costing $3 a bottle and $30 a bottle.[113] They are both labeled chondroitin, but one product is much better than the other.

Where those raw materials come from, how they are transported, where they are stored, and how they are processed can impact the potential quality. Did you realize that even supplements can contain metals and other toxins if they aren't high quality? There are fillers and binders that can be harmful. Fillers and binders bind the chemicals together in a particular supplement, and much like additives or dyes in food, they are common but can contain chemicals that can harm you over time. They can interfere with the active ingredients in the actual supplement and alter the supplement's digestion or absorption into the bloodstream.[114]

Even if you're trying to take care of yourself and do the right thing, you could be taking toxins into your system. I see this a lot with fitness buffs who go to the gym. They push themselves to the absolute limit, and then they drink all of these post-workout drinks and pop supplements without thinking twice about what's in them. If you look at all of the pre-workout, post-workout, weight-gain, weight-loss, and muscle-building supplements you take, many are loaded with chemicals, toxins, and even carcinogens.

Do you know what ingredients are in the supplements you're taking? From this point forward, try to make it a point to pay attention to what you put in your body. If you're taking these supplements, Google the ingredients to learn what they are. The higher-quality supplements have more quality ingredients with fewer chemicals, and ultimately that is what you're paying for. But with no universal standard, some companies and products are better than others, and how could you possibly know which supplements are the best to take?

REGULATION & OVERSIGHT

Since supplements aren't regulated by the FDA, quality varies significantly and there can be a lot of discrepancies between various brands, so you have to be careful. Given all the uncertainty surrounding supplements, some companies do their own independent quality control. Some have even taken it a step further by getting certification from those major bodies that regulate pharmaceuticals by getting certificates from:

- GMP – Good Manufacturing Practice.
- NSF International – Testing, auditing, and certification services.
- USP – Dietary Supplement Verification Program.
- TGA – Therapeutic Goods Administration (Australia).

Consumer Lab is another excellent resource that tracks and reports on the quality of the supplements on the market.[115] They are an independent lab that publishes a report every month. For $50 a year, you get access to the world of supplements and can see which companies got flagged, or just look up what individual companies claim is in their product versus what it actually contains. Believe it or not, there are many companies whose products don't live up to their own hype. This is a great resource that can protect the consumer.

FUN FACT:

The global dietary supplements market size was valued at $140.3 billion in 2020, and is expected to reach $272.4 billion by 2028.[116]

THE COMPANIES I RECOMMEND

Since I started my practice in 1998, I've always incorporated supplements, but we didn't have the technology we do today back then. I relied on a questionnaire, lab testing, and physical symptoms to determine a proper treatment plan. Data and resources were limited. Researching the products could take hours, but today there is more information, and there are more products than ever, so we face a different challenge. The supplement industry is growing rapidly, and new companies emerge all the time.

I'm always on the lookout for new suppliers and products. Often, my patients will bring a particular company to my attention. I'll do my research, and if it's an excellent product, I might recommend it. This is how I found a company called Elysium. A quick look at their advisory board revealed an impressive number of Nobel laureates and distinguished industry professionals, including one of my own professors at Stanford.[117] They focus on anti-aging products that I have gone on to recommend to patients.

It's not just important that you take supplements made by quality companies, but certain companies specialize in certain supplements. Smaller companies may focus on one or two, while larger companies have a wide array of supplements for all different conditions. The companies I recommend are the ones that go above and beyond the standards to ensure the best quality.

I've been doing this for 20 years and have challenged myself to study the latest products and technology. At my clinic, I give my patients supplements that typically have to be distributed by providers. Supplements in general don't require a prescription, but these are the closest to prescription-quality supplements because they have been analyzed and tested. They tend to be more potent, and in my experience, they lead to better results.

Everything I recommend is based on my experience. That includes what I've learned from research, seminars, experts, colleagues, and my own personal experience because I've tried them myself. I've checked the consumer lab report to make sure they haven't been flagged for any metals and toxins. I also talk with colleagues and other practitioners to get their opinion.

After compiling all of that data, a handful of companies have risen to the top and can be relied on to consistently provide a quality product. They all conduct third-party independent testing to ensure the purity of their ingredients. The sources and method of production are excellent. They may be more expensive, but consider it like buying a luxury car that simply performs better than the average functional car. These are the companies that stand out, and the ones I most frequently recommend:

- Metagenics
- Pure Encapsulations
- Vital Nutrients
- Orthomolecular Products
- Ayush Herbs
- Sun Potion
- Econugenics
- Jarrow Formulas
- Enviromedica
- Standard Process
- Integrative Therapeutics

Different companies specialize in different products. It just depends on what you're looking for. Hopefully my recommendations throughout the book help your decision making. As I always say to my patients, it's in your best interest to filter your mind, and filter your body for your life's sake. In other words it's important to screen what we hear, what we see and what we consume.

FUN FACT:

Three women were instrumental in the discovery of some key vitamins. Marguerite Davis co-discovered the existence of vitamin A in 1913. Katherine Bishop was part of the team that discovered vitamin E in 1922, and Lucy Wills was the sole discoverer of folic acid.[121]

THE CORE 8 SUPPLEMENTS

Since I've incorporated genomics in my practice, I've noticed some patterns. There are patterns in the way that we as Americans eat, there are patterns in the gene mutations I see in my patients, and there are patterns in the supplements I recommend that those patients take. Based on all of that, there are eight core supplements that I recommend my patients take for overall health and to help both treat and avoid the most common chronic conditions. These are the supplements that I believe everyone, regardless of age, gender, or overall health, can benefit from.

1. MULTI-VITAMINS

There is no one-size-fits-all multi-vitamin. It depends a lot on your age, gender, level of physical activity, and any underlying health conditions. Some of these are single doses with multiple pills, while others are available in chewable and powder forms. There are some excellent products out there, so it might require some trial and error when it comes to finding the multi-vitamin that is the best fit.

Recommended Products

- Metagenics – Wellness Essentials
- Pure Encapsulations – Nutrient 950

- Pure Encapsulations – Pure Genomics (helps address the most common mutations)
- Vital Nutrients – Multi-Nutrients

All of these products are excellent, high-end supplements, but the one I personally take and recommend to my patients is Wellness Essentials by Metagenics. It's important to note that this is more than a traditional multi-vitamin because it contains many of the other supplements on this core list, such as antioxidants, CoQ10, and fish oil, which is why a dose is six pills, which is also why it's the most expensive on the list. As a general rule, if a supplement makes you feel nauseous, you want to make sure you take it with food and consider splitting the dosage in half.

2. VITAMIN B12

B12 is a water-soluble vitamin that plays a role in energy production and methylation. It's a common ingredient in most multivitamins, but that doesn't mean you're taking the best version possible. According to expert Dr. Amy Yasko, since such a large portion of the population has an MTHFR mutation (or a mutation linked to methylation), the preferable form of B12 is adenosyl/hydroxy because it aids in methylation. Why not take the B12 that will help with you if you have a common mutation? Even if you don't have a mutation related to methylation, I believe that adenosyl/hydroxy is beneficial. It's similar to a higher-quality oil or gas for your car. Symptoms of a B12 deficiency can include fatigue, shortness of breath, and memory issues.[122]

Keep in mind that Vitamin B12 is crucial for those on a vegetarian or vegan diet, for this vitamin is not found in any plant products, which makes supplementation all the more important. You can get B12 from food sources such as shellfish, red meat, poultry, fish, eggs, milk, and cheese, but most people still fall significantly short of the recommended dosage, which is why supplementation is ideal.[123]

Recommended Products

- Pure Encapsulations
- Holistic Health

I personally take the liquid form of this supplement, so that I can put it in my smoothie or protein shake in the morning. Dr. Amy Yasko's supplement company, Holistic Health, was the first company to offer this adenosyl/hydroxy B12, and Pure Encapsulations followed, but very few other companies do, though that will most likely change because the demand is increasing.

NOTE: Caffeine can block the absorption of B-vitamins, and this includes coffee, so you want to take that into consideration when taking these supplements.

3. VITAMIN D3

Vitamin D isn't so much a vitamin as it is a hormone. It does so many things, including supporting bone, brain, muscle, and immune system function. A vitamin D deficiency can lead to numerous diseases, including osteoporosis.

Our skin also secretes vitamin D when exposed to the sunlight. However, just because you're out in the sun doesn't mean your body can properly absorb vitamin D. First, the body needs to break down vitamin D into vitamin D3, which is the absorbable form. This is a complex process that involves the parathyroid gland, kidneys, and the liver, so digestive issues, gut problems, poor diet, and lack of other vitamins and nutrients can all impair that process and ultimately lead to a vitamin D deficiency. This is the reason why many of my patients who live by the beach and are always out in the sun still suffer from vitamin D deficiencies.

I took Wellness Essentials, and even though it contains vitamin D, it wasn't enough to boost my levels into the preferred range. The normal range for vitamin D is 30 to 50 ng/mL, though I believe that 60 to 80 ng/mL is necessary for optimal function. When I started supplementing with a separate vitamin D3, it raised it into those ideal levels. It actually raised me above that level for a while, so I had to pull back. That's why it's always good to have your levels checked which most doctors and practitioners do these days as part of a standard panel.

Good food sources of vitamin D include fish liver oils, fatty fish, meats, milk, and certain dairy products.[124] However, medication such as anticonvulsant agents, barbiturates, cortisone, and mineral oil can impair fat absorption and decrease vitamin D's bioavailability.

The Significance of Vitamin D with K2

More and more products are offering vitamin D3 with K2. K2 is also getting a lot of attention, and just like vitamin D, many people are learning that their levels are low. One reason is because vitamin K is produced in the gut, and many people with intestinal issues have a deficiency. It supports the immune system, helps with inflammation, heart health, and bone health, and improves mood and absorption. However, vitamin K is also a blood-thinning supplement, so if you're already on blood-thinning medication, you want to speak with your primary care physician before adding K2. Vitamin K also serves an important function in that it binds to glutathione, which is a major antioxidant, and prevents it from becoming oxidized.

Recommended Products

- Vitamin D3 with K2 from Pure Encapsulations (liquid preferred).
- Vitamin D3 + K from Metagenics.
- Vitamin K2-7 + D3 from Vital Nutrients

Since vitamin D is made from an animal byproduct, Metagenics and Pure Encapsulations also have vegan versions.

FUN FACT:

According to some studies, post-menopausal women should take vitamin K2 to help with their bone mineral density, while reducing the potential for bone injuries and fractures.[125]

---

4. FISH OIL

The reason why I like fish oil so much is that it helps improve the health of your cells. Think of it as the protector of the cell and the cell membrane that houses and repairs the cell. The cell membrane is a barrier that shields the cell from the outside environment, but remains porous so material and nutrients can pass in and out when necessary. If the integrity of the membrane is jeopardized, the cell can be easily damaged, and with it, your DNA. And if the cell is damaged and doesn't function well, whatever organ or tissue it might be associated with also won't function well.

Let's say that the islets of Langerhans are damaged. For some reason this name stuck with me since 1995 when I attended chiropractic school; the islets of Langerhans are a cluster of cells within the pancreas that are responsible for the production and release of hormones, such as insulin and glucagon, that regulate the glucose levels in your blood. Insulin is the major hormone in the regulation of fat and protein metabolism. It's a crucial component of several metabolic processes. So damage to the isle of Langerhans' cells can lead to inadequate breakdown of carbohydrates, proteins, and fats, which can lead to inadequate single nutrients. This is how dysfunction at a cellular level in a specific location of an organ can affect our system as a whole and our DNA regulatory mechanisms. All of our cells and DNA rely on proper nutrition for healthy function and replication. Fish oil alone won't improve pancreatic issues, but it can improve cellular health and strengthen the cell membrane to prevent more serious issues from developing over time.

With fish oil, you definitely have to be careful. The problem is contamination and oxidation. You don't want to buy fish oil in plastic or clear bottles that have been exposed to the sun, because it will oxidize the oil quickly, and then it won't be as effective. That creates more free radicals. When purchasing fish oil, it's best that it comes in a dark glass bottle. Also be aware of where stores keep their products, because I have seen some stores put products like fish oil in their window display, directly in line with the sun.

WARNING: You want to be careful if you're on blood-thinning medication because fish oil, just like vitamin K, is a blood thinner as well, but otherwise, they are safe to take. [126]

Recommended Products

- Metagenics (as part of Wellness Essentials and as a single nutrient).
- Thorne – Omega Superb. (This is liquid and non-GMO.) Comes with Astaxanthin, rosemary extract, and is flavored with monk fruit. Also great for kids.)
- Pure Encapsulations.
- Orthomolecular Products – Orthomega – Mango (liquid and has a pleasant flavor).

The convenience of the Wellness Essentials multivitamin is that it also contains fish oil. If you're looking for a different source, Metagenics has about ten different kinds of fish oils for various conditions that include inflammation, arthritis, and oxidation. Given our diet in the United States, I typically lean toward supplements that help with inflammation since it can limit how the body functions and fish oil is an excellent anti-inflammatory.

FUN FACT:

According to a 2016 study in the New England Journal of Medicine, children whose mothers took fish oil supplements during pregnancy are less likely to develop asthma.[127]

---

5. PREBIOTICS

Think of the prebiotics like soil, and the probiotics are the seeds that need the soil to survive and thrive. If you have a condition like IBS, colitis, or Crohn's disease, they wipe out the soil, so the gut becomes like a barren desert.

The same can happen when you have to take antibiotics because they can impact your gut flora. But nobody's gut is perfect. We all have deficiencies.

Your gut is an open-ended system that keeps changing. It's been referred to as the second brain and your body's connection to the outside world, so it's important to keep it as healthy as possible. The gastrointestinal tract is made of microbes, and the integrity of those microbes is crucial when it comes to breaking down food and absorbing nutrients. Our knowledge about the microbiota in the gut continues to expand, and we keep learning there is much more to it than we thought.

Prebiotics are the non-digestible food ingredients that stimulate the growth of bacteria in the gut. When you think of prebiotics, you think of fructooligosaccharides (FOS). They improve your blood sugar levels and help fiber move more freely through your system. You can find FOS in garlic, leeks, artichokes, bananas, wheat, onions, asparagus, chicory, and various roots, but you have to consume such high quantities to get an adequate amount, which is why I recommend the supplements.[128]

I've been using prebiotics at my practice for years, and thankfully they are starting to get some attention as people realize their importance. More companies today are providing both prebiotics and probiotics.

Recommended Products:

- Metagenics – Probioplex Intensive Care (contains fructooligosaccharide, or FOS).
- Metagenics – Endefen (in powder form and contains arabinogalactans).
- Thorne – Effusio Prebiotic (comes in a water-dissolvable disc and has polyphenols/pomegranate fruit extract).
- Pure Encapsulations – Poly Prebiotic Powder (a combination of glucooligosaccharides and pomegranate fruit extract).

Don't forget that our gut is comprised of very diverse multi-functional, microbial inhabitants, so my advice is to rotate your prebiotics between the brands above.

6. PROBIOTICS

If the prebiotics are the soil, the probiotics are the live microorganisms (like seeds or live plants) that need that soil to thrive and inhibit the growth of pathogens. You can't have one without the other.

Probiotics have to make their way through the stomach and the small intestine to reach the large intestine, where they produce short-chain fatty acids from dietary fiber, maintain colonic pH, and prevent pathogens from adhering to the colonic mucosa, so they can eventually repopulate the colon. This usually requires six months of daily ingestion of 10 billion colony formula units, but certain gut conditions might require continued supplementation.[129]

The best way to check your gut health is through a DNA stool analysis, and the test I recommend is called GI Effects from Genova Diagnostics.[130] Thankfully, the technology of these tests has advanced as well. When I first started doing the stool test for my patients in the early 2000s, they had to collect their stool at home for three days and send it in. The test was still accurate, even though they had less information to work with when compared to today's tests.

Some foods are a good source of probiotics, particularly fermented foods like kimchi, sauerkraut, tempeh, kombucha, and low-sugar yogurt.

Recommended Products

- Metagenics
- Jarrow Formulas
- Pure Encapsulations
- Orthomolecular Products

Both Metagenics and Jarrow Formulas have numerous probiotic products based on various conditions such as immune health, gut balance, gut restore, and female hormone health. If you are concerned about immunity or often getting sick, I would recommend the Ultra Immune Booster from Metagenics. If you're frequently traveling, I would recommend UltraFlora Restore from Metagenics, or Orthomolecular Probiotic 225. It's also worth mentioning that Orthomolecular has a good children's line of probiotics. They have a few other supplements made specifically for kids, but these are limited.

NOTE: Prebiotics and probiotics can be taken together, but I recommend that you take your prebiotics separately and at different times than the probiotics. I personally believe it's better for absorption. It actually takes a lot for probiotics to be effective. First, they have to be digested, and then bypass the acid in your stomach to find the right area in your gut. If the prebiotics have done the work, the "soil" is ripe for them to flourish. Probiotics are best absorbed on an empty stomach. Some people take them in the morning, but I prefer to take them at night. Even if you take prebiotics and probiotics at different times during the day, there are numerous studies that have shown using both prebiotics and probiotics regularly has improved or prevented numerous gastrointestinal issues. It's referred to as some as microbiome therapy.[131]

7. FIBER

You usually get fiber from fruits and vegetables—some grains and nuts—but mainly fruits, vegetables, and legumes. The National Cancer Institute recommends 25 to 30 grams of fiber per day, depending on your sex and age. The preferred range is between 30 and 35 grams, but it's almost impossible to get all of that from fruits and vegetables alone. You have to eat bags and bags of kale, and that doesn't jibe with the standard diet, which is often comprised of meats, sweets, and sugar. Much like vitamin D or CoQ10, I've noticed that most people are deficient. When I do a dietary intake assessment for my patients, I find that most only eat 8 to 10 grams of fiber per day.

Soluble vs. Insoluble Fiber

Fiber helps with digestion and clearing out your system. It also lowers cholesterol because, as it moves through the gut, it picks up those molecules and helps the body excrete them. It lowers blood sugar and is an immune stimulant. But there are so many different types of fiber out there. Which one is right for you? It can be overwhelming when trying to pick out the right product, especially when you consider that people can have reactions to certain products. Sometimes, you can't really tell what type of response you will have until you try it.

One useful distinction to make when choosing a fiber is if you would benefit from soluble or insoluble. The main difference is that, as the name implies, the insoluble fiber doesn't break apart. It has more of a laxative effect that keeps everything moving through your digestive tract. Soluble fiber does break apart more easily, so it helps aid in digestion, lower blood sugar, and lower blood insulin levels.[132] Soluble fiber adds some bulk and softness to the stools because of the way it absorbs water, and also increases that feeling of fullness after eating.

Here are some examples of each:

- Insoluble fiber: Celluloses, lignins, some hemicelluloses.
- Soluble fibers: Pectins, gums, mucilages, alginates, carrageenans, some hemicelluloses.

Recommended Products

- Orthomolecular Products – Fiber Plus
- Metagenics — MetaFiber

So many clients ask me about name-brand fibers they can buy at the store, and I tell them to Google the ingredients, and then write "unhealthy" or carcinogen" at the end of each ingredient. Try it and see what comes up.

NOTE: You want to take fiber on its own and on an empty stomach, because it can block the absorption of other supplements and nutrients. I recommend that you take it either in the morning or at night. I chose to take it at night, but if you do take it in the morning, you should wait at least an hour before taking other vitamins, especially B vitamins. Keep in mind that it can be difficult for some people to take fiber, so plan accordingly by starting slowly and gradually increasing the amount. While you increase your fiber intake, you also want to increase your water intake to avoid bowl obstruction and constipation. And you will know if you're taking too much fiber with water if you experience diarrhea.

8. ANTIOXIDANTS

When your body breaks down food or is exposed to toxins, it produces free radicals, which can break DNA's double-strand bonds. If not repaired, that can lead to cell death, genomic instability, disease, and other acute and chronic conditions. Antioxidants protect your cells from those free radicals by making the molecules more stable, so the body can more easily remove them. This is another reason why the detox is so important; but in today's world, your body tends to always accumulate more toxins and free radicals, so consuming antioxidants is a good way to keep them at a minimum while maintaining your cellular health even after the detox.

When you get your DNA raw data, you'll see that there are over 50 genes related to the Cytochrome P450 pathway, determining how well your body removes toxins and your antioxidant function.[133] If you see a lot of red and yellow in that report, it means that your system needs help, and you are a prime candidate for antioxidant supplements; but antioxidants are something everyone can benefit from. There is a wide range of antioxidants, and you want to take more than one source, so here is a list of the major ones to focus on:

*Glutathione: Often called nature's "master antioxidant," this major cellular antioxidant is composed of cysteine, glutamine, and glycine. You can take in supplement form that helps with all kinds of toxins. It stabilizes your immune system and helps the liver function better, but it also decreases as we age. We can get this antioxidant from food sources like meat, poultry, fish, soy, corn, nuts, milk, and cheese, but rarely is it enough. It's also possible to have a mutation in the GSTT1 gene, which can limit the amount of glutathione you produce and make it difficult for your body to naturally remove toxins. If you have this mutation, you would want to take a glutathione supplement for the rest of your life. Deficiency may result in oxidative stress, impaired detoxification, immune deficiency, macular degeneration, significantly increased risk of hypertension, and increased risk of carcinomas.

- *Recommended Products*

▷ Liposomal Glutathione from Pure Encapsulations (pills and liquid).

▷ Metagenics – GlutaClear.

*CoQ10: This powerful antioxidant is synthesized in the body and contained in the cell membrane. When talking about CoQ10, we're talking about energy production and pH regulation. It also helps with the oxidation of the cell and protects DNA from oxidative stress. Without oxygen, there is no life or cellular health, and if you are low on CoQ10, your cells won't get enough oxygen. Deficiencies in CoQ10 can occur because of statins, diabetic medication, and heart medication (beta-blockers). That can result in oxidative stress, diabetes, cancer, congestive heart failure, cardiac arrhythmias, gingivitis, and neurologic disease.[134] Since your cells replicate every few months, you want to make sure that the cell template is intact so that the organ or system won't suffer. We can get CoQ10 in our diet from food sources like meat, fish, poultry, soybean, canola oil, nuts, and whole grains. Moderate sources can come from fruit, vegetables, eggs, and dairy. There's a lot that CoQ10 does. In addition to energy and fatigue, some people take it for anti-aging. I take it for heart health, since I have a history of cardiovascular disease on my dad's side of the family, and inherited some of those genes. This is an important supplement because six out of the ten people I test for CoQ10 have very low levels.

- *Recommended Products*
    ▷ Metagenics – CoQ10 ST.
    ▷ Thorne – Q-Best 100.
    ▷ Ayush Herbs – CoCurcumin CoQ10 – This comes in powder form and combines high-quality curcumin and CoQ10 with medium-chain triglycerides (MCTs), which improves the bioavailability and absorption of curcumin and CoQ10.

*NAC: This supplement boosts antioxidant function and raises glutathione levels to help support the body's response to inflammation. It can also clear sinus congestion while supporting respiratory and pulmonary health, which makes it a good supplement to take when sick with the flu. It protects the body from oxidative damage, enhances detoxification, and aids in the breakdown of toxins. NAC is worth looking into because it can help improve energy, immunity, and cellular health, and even aid in preventing conditions and diseases. I like NAC because it's the master regulator against inflammation. Think of it like a switch that controls inflammation. It also helps aid in stress, cardiovascular health, oncology support, energy, and immunity.[135] One supplement that works well with NAC is lipoic acid. Just keep in mind that these NAC supplements can be a very expensive product that ranges from $120 to $140 per bottle.

- *Recommended Product*
  - ▷ Orthomolecular Products — N-Acetyl Cysteine (NAC)

*Plant-Based Antioxidants: When it comes to antioxidants, you also want to think of green vegetables: the darker the greens, the more antioxidant protection you get. That's why fruits and vegetables are excellent sources of antioxidants, but the problem is that you have to eat such large quantities to get the necessary levels of antioxidants in your diet. It's so much easier to take a scoop of powder.

- *Recommended Products*
  - ▷ Orthomolecular Products – Indigo Greens.
  - ▷ Metagenics – Oxygenics (cellular mitochondria support for energy that includes CoQ10, NAC, and other antioxidants together).
  - ▷ Metagenics – PhytoGanix.

*L-Carnitine: This antioxidant helps break down fat by directing the source of fuel to come from fat cells instead of from carbohydrates and protein. It can help aid in in the treatment of heart disease, mental performance, liver disease, and weight loss.

- ▷ Pure Encapsulations – CoQ10 L-Carnitine Fumarate.
- ▷ Vital Nutrients – Carnitine.
- ▷ Metagenics – L-Carnitine.

*Alpha Lipoic Acid: In addition to being an antioxidant that plays an essential role in mitochondrial dehydrogenase reactions—which are critical for cell processes and keeping our body's systems in balance—it protects the body from oxidative stress and the conditions that can develop as a result. Alpha lipoic acid also breaks down carbohydrates to create energy for other organs in the body, while lowering blood sugar and eliminating free radicals.[136]

> ▷ Pure Encapsulations – Alpha Lipoic Acid (comes in different strengths and is non-GMO, gluten free, vegan, and vegetarian).
> ▷ Metagenics – Meta Lipoate 300.
> ▷ Thorne – Alpha-Lipoic Acid (single nutrient).
> ▷ Thorne – Diabenil (in addition to Alpha Lipoic Acid it offers comprehensive support for healthy blood sugar levels).
> ▷ Vital Nutrient – Alpha Lipoic Acid (single nutrient).

*Vitamin E: This is the body's main fat-soluble antioxidant and an essential nutrient. Vitamin E is important because of the large quantity of fat we consume daily. It improves mitochondrial function (think of cellular energy) and immune function, while stopping the production of ROS when fat undergoes oxidation. There is evidence to suggest it can help prevent or delay the diseases associated with free radicals.[137] Usually a good multivitamin will cover your needs for Vitamin E, but if needed as a single nutrient, I highly recommend the following products.

> ▷ Pure Encapsulations – Vitamin E.
> ▷ Vital Nutrients – Natural Vitamin E (this is free of coatings, binders, gluten, milk, dairy, egg protein, and sugar, but does contain soy).
> ▷ Pure Encapsulations – Q-Gel 100 (combines a ready-to-absorb highly soluble CoQ10 with Vitamin E. It's also non GMO).

*DIM/I3C: I3C (Indole 3 carbinol) is found in cruciferous vegetables like broccoli and Brussels sprouts. I3C is converted to DIM, and even though DIM and I3C are different molecules with different chemical structures, they function in a similar way. Supplementing with DIM supports hormone detoxification and estrogen balance and metabolism for men and women.

> ▷ Thorne – Indole-3-Carbinol
> ▷ Pure Encapsulations – Indole-3-Carbinol

▷ Metagenics – Meta I3C

FUN FACT:

Where you keep your supplements is important. Storing them in humid places, like the bathroom or kitchen, where they might be subjected to steam, and heat can degrade the effectiveness of the ingredients. As the saying goes: store in a cool, dry place.[138]

CONDITION-SPECIFIC SUPPLEMENTS

*L-Theanine: This amino acid helps with anxiety, stress, and sleep. You can take multiple doses throughout the day or in a moment when you need to feel calm. It can be effective and in a way that leaves you alert and not groggy, jittery, or in need of a stimulant, so you can still function, even if you increase the dosage. I've had patients say that it gives them a euphoric feeling and energy that combats fatigue. It is becoming a popular product. I even saw an energy drink that contained L-theanine that was probably added to counteract the jittery effect from the caffeine and other ingredients. However, you have to be careful if you're taking antidepressants or stimulant medications, because it might affect the medication.[139]

Recommended Supplementation

- Vital Nutrients: L-Theanine
- Thorne: Theanine

*5HTP: This helps increase serotonin synthesis, which can influence sleep, appetite, and sexual function. This can help aid in the prevention of depression, insomnia, and obesity. 5HTP is very similar to what an SSRI medication does. SSRI stands for "selective serotonin reuptake inhibitor." However, you have to be careful and should consult your primary care physician if you're taking antidepressants or stimulants, because it might affect the medication.

Recommended Supplementation

- Thorne: 5-Hydroxytryptophan
- Orthomolecular Products: 5HTP
- Pure Encapsulations: 5 HTP

*SAMe – This helps with brain neurotransmitters, which means it can aid in conditions like depression, anxiety, high cholesterol, and PMS while raising homocysteine levels. It can work well, but you want to be careful with SAMe, and its use should be supervised because it can lead to nausea, digestive problems, and exacerbate other issues. It also SHOULD NOT be used with antidepressants or diabetes medication.[140]

Recommended Supplementation

- Orthomolecular Products: SAMe
- Pure Encapsulations: SAMe

*Molybdenum – This is an excellent supplement that helps process sulfur reaction, oxidation, and is also good for anti-aging. It can be found in meat, cereals, peas, and beans. Chronic deficiency may limit life expectancy and reproduction.[141] This aids in the detoxification of sulfite and supplementation is beneficial in those with a sensitivity to sulfite. I personally like this supplement better as a single nutrient and have seen people experience speedy results.

Recommended Supplementation

- Thorne: Molybdenum Glycinate
- Pure Encapsulations: As part of "Trace Minerals," which is one of my go-to supplements for trace mineral supplementation.

*Selenium: An essential antioxidant, selenium is a cofactor of glutathione peroxidase and works with vitamin E that helps to combat free radicals and infection. Often found in meat and seafood, it also aids in reproduction, thyroid gland function, immune function, and DNA production. Selenium deficiency can lead to decreased immunity protection, cardiovascular issues, increased inflammation, thyroid issues, and male and female reproductive health issues. It is believed that selenium supplementation can help reduce the risk of some cancers because of its ability to repair DNA. With selenium, it's important to rotate between different forms, such as selenomethionine, citrate sodium selenite, selenium L-aspartate, and chelate. Please be advised that high intakes of selenium can be toxic. I follow the age appropriate daily upper limit guidelines for selenium set by the National Institute of Health (NIH).

Recommended Supplementation

- Vital Nutrients: Selenium.
- Pure Encapsulations: Selenium citrate.
- Thorne: Selenomethionine.
- Metagenics: E400 Selenium.
- Orthomolecular Products: Reacted Selenium.

*Garlic: Garlic contains allicin and allylic sulfides, which can reduce cholesterol and blood pressure, and increase resistance to infectious organisms and parasites. Garlic does so many different things. It's an immune booster, anti-microbial, anti-viral, anti-inflammatory, and helps prevent clogging of the arterial walls. However, you want to take garlic by itself because it's powerful and may overpower other immune stimulants you're taking. I personally take garlic and have experienced the benefits. Garlic is unique in that it is also a spice, and I take both—garlic in supplement form, and frequently use the spice when cooking. As with most all of my spices, I get my garlic from a company called Frontier Co-Op.

Recommended Supplementation

- Metagenics: Super Garlic 6000. I've been taking this supplement for years now on an empty stomach upon waking up with no issues because of its special enteric coating, which is designed to dissolve in the intestine.

MINERALS & ELECTROLYTES

*Magnesium: This mineral is a major component of bones and teeth, and necessary for muscle relaxation. If you're taking any diuretics, they can deplete magnesium. A magnesium deficiency can lead to hyperthyroidism, cramps, nausea, irritability, and cardiac arrhythmias. Supplementing with magnesium may improve insulin resistance, hypertension, muscle cramps, and bone mineral density. It's important to rotate between the different forms of magnesium, which include magnesium, citrate, bisglycinate, malate, glycinate, aspartate, L-threonate, oxide, chelate, lysinate, and lactate.

Recommended Supplementation

- Metagenics: Mag L-Threonate.
- Vital Nutrients: Triple Mag.
- Pure Encapsulations: UltraMag (there are various forms, including liquid and powder).
- Thorne: Various forms.
- Orthomolecular Products: Reacted Magnesium Powder.
- Standard Process: Magnesium Lactate.

You want to be careful with magnesium, because there are some risk factors and side effects. Magnesium can interact with some antibiotics, diuretics, and heart medications. If you have diabetes, intestinal disease, heart disease, and kidney disease, you should consult with your physician before taking magnesium. You know you've taken too much if you experience nausea, diarrhea, low blood pressure, weakness, or fatigue. It can even be deadly, so you definitely want to be careful.

*Calcium: All calcium is stored in bones and teeth, where it supports their structure. Calcium is essential for making muscles move and for nerves to transmit messages throughout the body. When your calcium levels are low, your body takes it from your bones, decreasing their density and making them weak and brittle. You want to rotate between the different forms of calcium, such as hydroxyapatite, di-calcium malate, glycinate, chelate, glucarate, citrate, and lactate.

Recommended Supplementation

- Orthomolecular Products (various forms).
- Metagenics (various forms).
- Vital Nutrients (various forms).

- Pure Encapsulations (various forms).
- Thorne (various forms).
- Standard Process (various forms).

Calcium is another mineral you have to be careful with. Even if you take normal doses, you may experience gas, bloating, and constipation. Take too much and it can cause kidney stones, irregular heartbeat, confusion, and even death. There is some conflicting data, but some studies show that diets high in calcium can increase your risk of heart attack and stroke. High doses can prevent your body from absorbing iron and zinc, and it's a good idea to take it two hours apart from other medication and supplements. Keep in mind that high doses of vitamin D can raise calcium levels. And always check with your physician because calcium can also interact with some prescription medication, and cause complications if you have kidney disease, heart problems, sarcoidosis, or bone tumors.

*Chloride: This is one of the most important electrolytes as it keeps your blood and bodily fluids in balance. High chloride levels could indicate kidney problems, while low chloride levels are most often involved with vomiting and dehydration. Congestive heart failure (when your heart muscle is weakened and can't pump enough blood to your body) is one of the most serious diseases associated with low chloride levels. Chloride is often included as part of a trace mineral supplement, but the following products are also good sources.

Recommended Supplementation

- Standard Process: Cal-Amo in combination with calcium.
- Pure Encapsulations: Multi-Mineral Liquid.

*Phosphorus: In addition to being a component of bone structure, phosphorus regulates energy metabolism and plays a crucial role in how the body uses carbohydrates and fats. Phosphorus also aids in the creation of protein to grow and repair cells and tissues. It's rare to have low levels of phosphorus, since you can find it in so many different foods. Low levels often occur in cases of starvation, alcoholism, chronic use of aluminum-base antacids, and eating disorders. High levels are associated with chronic kidney disease and increase your risk of heart attack and stroke. Diarrhea and stomach cramps are often an indication that you're taking too much. Phosphorus is often part of mineral/trace element support supplements, but the following product is also a good source.

Recommended Supplementation

- Orthomolecular Products: Reacted MultiMin. Includes broad-spectrum mineral support.

*Potassium: A major intracellular electrolyte, potassium helps muscles contract and aids in nerve function. It helps move nutrients into cells while removing necessary waste. Your kidneys help to regulate potassium levels, but some medication can raise those levels. You want to rotate between the different forms of potassium, such as citrate, aspartate, iodide, and glycinate. The following brands are all great sources for potassium, and they all have various forms and combinations. Most are sold as potassium and magnesium supplements together.

Recommended Supplementation

- Orthomolecular Products
- Metagenics
- Vital Nutrients
- Pure Encapsulations
- Thorne

If you take too much potassium, you risk serious cardiovascular concerns, and you might experience irregular heartbeat, confusion, tingling limbs, low blood pressure, muscle weakness, and even muscle paralysis or coma. If you suffer from kidney disease, heart disease, Addison's disease, stomach ulcers or other medical conditions, you should speak with your physician before taking any potassium supplements.

*Sodium: Both a mineral and an electrolyte, sodium regulates extracellular fluid volume. Most commonly found in salt, sodium contributes to how nerves and muscles work. Too much sodium can increase blood pressure and cause your body to retain fluids. That can possibly result in numerous conditions such as kidney disease and stroke.

CAPSULE, TABLET, POWDER, OR LIQUID?

Before purchasing any supplement, it's important to consider the source and the form because that plays a vital role. Supplements are made from different sources, such as natural, plant derived, food based, through bacterial fermentation, and synthetic. You typically have four different options when shopping for supplements based on their size, shape, and rigidity:

- Capsule
- Tablet
- Powder
- Liquid

CAPSULES

Capsules are made from gelatin or vegetable cellulose (vegan/vegetarian option). Gelatin is more widely used by the supplement industry because its benefits may include help with digestion, providing joint protection and joint pain relief, and improving sleep. Unless they are practitioner-grade supplements, caution must be exercised for toxic metal contamination due to variation in gelatin production during pretreatment, extraction, and refining.

Pros:

- Easily opened and mixed into a smoothie or another powdered supplement
- Usually there is no aftertaste
- Capsule-filling options include liquid or powder form
- Liquid-filled capsules are easily absorbed by our digestive tract, usually within minutes

Cons:

- Capsule content inconsistencies due to volume variations
- Tend to be more expensive

TABLETS

Most tablets are made from compressed powdered ingredients. They come in two forms, either coated (usually with sugar) or uncoated. Most often the absorption rate is within twenty to thirty minutes.

Pros:

- Most nutrient packed
- Can be crushed into powder and mixed in a smoothie or another powdered supplement
- Chewable tablet options are a great alternative for children or adults who have difficulty swallowing pills
- More affordable
- Longer shelf life

Cons:

- Sugar coating
- Longer absorption rate than capsules or liquid supplements
- Potential for more additives, especially with Non-Practioner Grade supplements

POWDER

Various processes of extracting, drying, and filtering the nutrients are implemented to make powder supplements.

Pros:

- Dosage can be easily adjusted
- Longer shelf life
- Great alternative for children or adults who have difficulty swallowing pills
- Easily mixed with water, smoothies, or other powdered supplements
- Easily digested

Cons:

- Powders may contain added sugars for flavoring

- Process variations of extracting, drying, and filtering may reflect powder quality

Liquid

Liquids are often made from products that are either natural, plant derived, or synthetic, and may have added flavors.

Pros:

- High absorption rate, usually within one to four minutes
- Easily digested
- High potency rate
- Great alternative for children or adults who have difficulty swallowing pills
- Flexible dosage

Cons:

- May contain added sugars for flavoring
- Refrigeration may be required
- Not travel friendly
- Shorter shelf life
- Taste and smell may vary
- May include harmful additives such as hydrogenated oils, boric acid, and sodium benzoate, especially with Non-Practioner Grade supplements

In addition to the different types mentioned above, supplements may also be categorized based on their absorption rate and when and where they are released in our gastrointestinal tract. Below is a brief explanation of each subcategory.

- ENTERIC COATED: supplements that bypass the stomach first before releasing their active nutrients into the intestines.
- SUSTAINED RELEASE: supplements that release their ingredients into the digestive tract over an extended period of time rather than all at once.
- LIPOSOMAL: supplements that are encapsulated in fat cells called liposomes, which help improve their absorption rate. They

are made of the same material as our cell membranes (cell's gate keeper). Therefore, their nutrients are transported directly into the cells of our tissues, enhancing their absorption and bioavailability rate.

In general, all supplement options are good, and different forms have pros and cons. However, there remains a possibility of a dietary supplement to be contaminated with heavy metals unless they are Practitioner Grade supplements. As always do your research, be mindful of what you are taking, and talk to your doctor before adding supplements to your diet.

Liquid is the most difficult form to keep stable, which is why it is often the most expensive option, but it is also the easiest for the body to absorb, along with liposomal supplements, so that is why I always recommend my patients look into a liquid supplement first before considering other options. It is also easier and more convenient to take liquid supplements. Some people struggle swallowing pills, and some of these supplements are giant horse pills, but with a liquid, you can put it in your morning shake or protein drink. Liquid supplements are also ideal if you have gut issues, because they are the easiest to absorb. Whether it is supplements or nutrition, iti s all about absorption and how well your gut is functioning. That' s why the detox is so important.

HOW MUCH WILL THIS COST ME?

The reality is that quality supplements can be expensive. If you were to take just the core supplements listed here, you're looking at $150 to $200 a month. Not everyone can make that kind of investment. If you need to prioritize, start with the Wellness Essentials. Then incorporate the adenosyl/ hydroxy B-12 and probiotics, because gut health is so important.

There are short-term benefits and long-term benefits. Those patients who experienced low energy or low testosterone can sometimes see an immediate effect. Those patients who are already healthy might not notice any immediate short-term benefits, but they will most definitely experience long-term benefits, as would most anyone else taking quality supplements.

However, it's easier to stop taking supplements or opt for the less expensive (lower-quality) alternatives if you aren't experiencing those short-term or immediate results. It becomes a personal choice, but as I said initially, you get what you pay for when it comes to supplements. There isn't a shortcut.

If you're just venturing into the world of supplementation, take it slow. It's easy to go overboard. You want to take it easy and not overtax the liver. Do everything in moderation and pay attention to your genetics. You don't want to take supplements just to take them. Take only the supplements that you need.

FUN FACT:

The dietary supplement industry provides more than 383,000 quality jobs in the United States—paying over $18 billion in wages each year.[143]

START SLOWLY

After the detox, your liver goes through a significant cleansing. Do it properly, and it's like you finish the detox with practically a brand-new organ. Not only does the detox reset the liver, but also the way organs, systems, and neurotransmitters work. You don't want to begin taking other supplements at the start of the detox. But during those final days of the detox, your absorption levels are really top-notch, so that's why when my patients begin to reduce the shakes and reintroduce some of their everyday foods once again, I start them on a supplement regimen. Do it slowly. You don't want to overwhelm your system, but plan it out ahead of time.

DON'T EVER GET TOO COMFORTABLE

The human body is complex. It's very smart, and it can adapt exceptionally well. For those who exercise frequently or go to the gym, you probably know that you have to switch up your workout routine to avoid plateauing. The same is true for supplements. Your body can adapt to certain brands and supplement routines, so after some time, you're no longer maximizing the product's effectiveness. That's why I recommend people rotate supplement brands. These bottles and packages usually come in 30-day or 60-day supplies. Simply purchase a quality product from a different source when the first one runs out. If you have two or three sources for each product, that's a solid rotation, so your body won't adapt and the supplement can continue to be effective.

FUN FACT:

Technology continues to advance, and there is no reason to think that the supplement industry won't be positively impacted as well. It's possible that supplements of the future will involve gut microbes, genetic coding, and other personalized features to make them more effective.[144]

HOW DO I KNOW IF THIS IS WORKING?

I've said it before, but everyone is different. We all start from a different place. We suffer from different conditions and have a different genome with different mutations. What worked for someone else may not work as quickly or as well for you.

If you're someone who is already experiencing physical symptoms—lack of energy, fatigue, or stress—then you have an excellent chance of experiencing relief. As soon as I added the Wellness Essentials, the B12, and vitamin D to my regimen, I personally noticed that I handled stress better and had more energy.

Deborah, one of my patients, loved to travel but suffered from arthritis and other symptoms that prevented her from enjoying the experience. She had to sit out some tour groups, and other days she couldn't leave the hotel because of aches and pains. We put her through the detox and then gave her supplements based on her genes. After a few months, she felt better, looked younger, and even lost weight. When she resumed traveling, she was able to participate in everything. It made that much of a difference.

If you're taking a supplement because of a genetic mutation for which you aren't experiencing symptoms, you may not notice any immediate difference, but know that you can still experience benefits by preventing a possible condition from developing down the road. Down the road can arrive quicker than you think. When you pass 40, you start to feel different. By 50, it becomes more urgent.

You don't only have to go by how you feel. If you have the resources, I recommend that you get your blood work done every six months, because a lot of things can happen over the course of an entire year, and it's better to catch any issues early. I also recommend more comprehensive functional medicine lab tests. Many used to cost a couple thousand dollars, and now they are only a couple hundred. One of my go-to tests for a complete nutritional evaluation is called NutrEval from Genova Diagnostics.[145] They take insurance but also have a cash price. It's a comprehensive test that measures all the vitamins and amino acids in your system. If that isn't an option, I recommend that you test the fat-soluble vitamins (like vitamin D, vitamin A vitamin K, CoQ10) because they tend to accumulate over time and become toxic.

FULLSCRIPT

Technology has advanced now to the point that my patients can get the products that I recommend from almost every company shipped directly to their house through a service called Fullscript. This is a free, Practitioner - Grade online supplement dispensary for practitioners. This can take the place of in-office dispensaries. From this site, I can monitor patient refills and provide recommendations. Many practitioners do the same thing, because it's more efficient, and it saves time. You can take advantage of this for yourself by going to my own website to purchase supplements: https://www.drmichaelswellness.com/store.

You may also purchase Metagenics products directly from my website. I will have all the products we mentioned in the book available.

For Metagenics products, visit this link:

https://mmichael.metagenics.com

For all other products, visit FullScript at this link:

https://us.fullscript.com/welcome/mmichael

METAGENICS

FULLSCRIPT

CHAPTER 7:

A NEW APPROACH TO FITNESS
AND WORKING OUT

WHEN IT COMES TO EPIGENETICS AND OUTSIDE FACTORS THAT CAN CAUSE a protein in certain genes to express (basically turning those genes on and off), nutrition, supplementation, and environmental factors all play a role. Another major factor is exercise.

Fitness and exercise are broad categories that mean different things to different people. Everyone is starting from a different point and faces different challenges when it comes to fitness, so there is no one-size-fits-all approach to how you incorporate fitness into your daily life. A 70-year-old woman will have a much different regimen than a 25-year-old man, but they can each be healthy and fit—they just have to go about it in a different way. However, if you live a more sedentary life, it can be a challenge to break the routine, create a new habit, and get started. However, there are a few tricks that can help you begin a fitness and exercise routine if you find yourself having trouble getting active.

1. *Walking*

That's it. Just walk. Anybody can benefit from walking, no matter what their age. The benefits of walking have been very well studied, and it has been shown to have a direct positive effect on cardiovascular health, longevity, and overall well-being.[146] If you're older and you're not used to going to the gym, you don't want to suddenly go to the gym out of the blue because you might end up getting hurt. It's not that I believe that older people aren't capable, but when you get hurt, it can set you back. Depending on the individual, an injury might discourage that person from even trying.

At first, keep it simple, and it doesn't get any simpler than walking. As you progress, you can take advantage of long and slow distance training, or what I like to call "conversational walking." This is walking at a fast pace—a maximum of 70 percent of your oxygen capacity—for anywhere between 30 minutes and two hours. The idea is to walk at brisk pace, but not so fast that you aren't able to talk. This type of exercise helps with cardiovascular function, improves energy production, and helps the body break down fat by utilizing it as fuel.[147]

2. Do What You Love

One trick is to zero in on hobbies, so if there is something you like to do that is fitness-related, try to do more of it. If you like to bike, and do it once or twice a week, try increasing that to three or four times a week. If you've done something in the past, it's so much easier to keep doing that thing than it is to incorporate a completely different activity. Just give yourself a little extra push. And if you decide to stop doing a particular exercise or activity, make sure you replace it with another. That's a process that I call "activity periodization."

3. Take Advantage of Online Classes

Since the pandemic, there are more programs and classes online than ever before. You don't even have to leave your house. Peloton offers classes, as do many local gyms and clubs, so you can take various yoga and fitness classes. You don't even have to belong to a gym, you can go on YouTube and find hundreds of workouts that you can do from your house. There are so many possibilities out there that you might not even know about until you look. My neighbor teaches karate online. I didn't even know you could do that until he told me. Since then, I started taking Krav Maga classes online. The key is to have the motivation and the time, so if you're a person who struggles with exercise, start small with something you can easily incorporate into your daily routine to create a habit, and then build on that habit.

Exercise helps with your mental health and overall brain chemistry by stimulating parts of your brain that aren't responsive when you're depressed by releasing endorphins, a neurotransmitter that helps to relieve pain and stress. Exercise also releases dopamine, norepinephrine, and serotonin, which all help to regulate your mood. These are feel-good hormones that can give you a feeling like a runner's high. That feeling is addictive, but it's a good addiction to have because it will help you think better, feel better, and handle stress better. The CDC recommends getting 150 minutes of aerobic activity a week, and that includes walking, swimming, biking, rowing, or playing a sport like basketball.[148]

FUN FACT:
A 2010 study shows that listening to music while exercising can delay fatigue and increase work capacity, leading to higher-than-expected levels of endurance, power, productivity, and strength. Music is also believed to distract from the pain endured during exercise.[149]

THE ATHLETE GENE

The reason my wife was able to get better results faster, and experience greater benefit from the same exact exercise, was because of the ACTN3 gene. What this gene does is encode proteins present in fast-twitch muscle fibers. On average, people have about 50 percent fast-twitch muscle fibers and 50 percent slow-twitch, but this gene can determine if you have more of one type or another. What's the difference?

- SLOW-TWITCH MUSCLE FIBERS (Type I) – These fibers are slower to contract and smaller in diameter. They have more oxidative enzymes, mitochondria, and capillaries, which lead to higher aerobic function and a higher resistance to fatigue. In other words, they fire slowly, and have extended muscle contraction, which leads to high endurance. Most marathon runners tend to have this type of muscle fiber.[150]

- FAST-TWITCH MUSCLE FIBERS (Type II) – These are responsible for movements and exercises that require quick bursts, such as sprinting, jumping and explosive movements. They provide short bursts of speed, but also fatigue quicker. They use both fat and glycogen for energy. Most sprinters tend to have this type of muscle fiber, as do bodybuilders, since fast-twitch muscle fibers play a significant role in muscle growth.

There are even two types of fast-twitch muscle fibers, non-oxidative and oxidative-glycolytic, and there are hybrid forms as well. For many movements and exercises you use both types. Here is an example of the involvement of both slow and fast twitch muscle fibers in the following spots, events, and lifts.

Event:	Slow Twitch	Fast Twitch:
100-meter sprint	Low	High
800-meter run	High	High
Marathon	High	Low
Olympic weightlifting	Low	High
Barbell Squat	High	High
Soccer	High	High
Field hockey	High	High
Football WR	Low	High
Football lineman	High	High
Basketball	Low	High
Distance cycling:	High	Low[151]

Not only does your muscle fiber type impact what type of activities you're better suited for, but it also impacts how you train, and the effectiveness of your workout. Those with fast-twitch muscle fibers benefit more from a style of exercise that resembles circuit training, or plyometric exercises with quick bursts, like box jumps, sprints, squats, and bench presses. Those with low-twitch muscle-fibers benefit from more endurance activities like swimming, cycling, and long-distance running.

If my wife and I went to the gym and wanted to go through a leg workout, we would each benefit from a different approach. Since I have more slow-twitch muscle fibers, I would do a more traditional workout with four or five sets of squats (and two or three minutes in between each set) before moving onto the next exercise. My wife would benefit more from supersets or circuit training programs. So, she would do one set of squats and then immediately move onto the next exercise to do a set, and the next exercise to do a set without resting. One set each of multiple exercises would be one full set for her.

Just because you have more of a certain type of muscle fiber doesn't mean that you can only benefit from these exercises. As long as you do the exercise, the benefit is there, but you can improve the way your body responds, and see greater results if you work out according to your genes.

About 80 percent of people have at least one functioning copy of the ACTN3 gene. The remaining 20 percent may have significantly less strength, speed, and athleticism. That doesn't mean that those in this group can't succeed in sports or lead healthy lifestyles, but they might have to work out differently, perhaps even harder, especially if they are competing in sports that favor those with the ACTN3 gene.

FUN FACT:

The more muscle mass you have, the more fat you burn, even when at rest. According to one Wharton study, 10 pounds of muscle would burn 50 calories in a day at rest, while 10 pounds of fat would burn only 20 calories.[152]

GENES AND YOUR PERFORMANCE

One version of the ACTN3 gene has been found in almost every Olympic sprinter ever tested, but still, it's just one of many genes that contribute to athleticism. Genetics have a significant influence over strength, muscle size, lung capacity, flexibility, anaerobic threshold, and endurance.

*EDN1 – This mutation can increase hypertension in those with poor cardiovascular fitness.

*LPL – There has been a link between this gene and the ability to lose body fat during exercise.

*LIPC – This gene has been linked to insulin sensitivity in response to exercise.

*PLXNA4 – A mutation in this gene increases your risk of concussion.

*VHL – This gene is part of what helps cells survive when oxygen is reduced. A mutation can limit one's aerobic exercise capacity.[153]

*MSTN – Unusual muscle size and strength is often a result of this gene.

*IL15RA – This gene is linked to the prevention of muscle breakdown and how quickly you can increase muscle size. Some experience increases in strength with less muscle size, and others experience the opposite.

*IGF1 & IGF1_2 – These are two more genes that influence muscle growth and development.

*MCT1 – Do you get fatigued easily when you exercise? That might be because of this gene, which leads to slow clearing of lactic acid in the muscles.

*IL6 – This gene controls inflammation, and a higher expression can lead to lower BMI and endurance, while a lower expression can lead to weight gain and slow recovery.

*PGC1A – This is an aerobic capacity gene. It allows your body to work harder during long bouts of exercise.

*CKM – How energy is used and how you process oxygen are impacted by this gene.

*UCP2 – This is linked to faster metabolism and a lower risk of weight gain.

*UCP3 – This gene is associated with a lower metabolic rate and an inefficient metabolism, so you are more likely to have a greater BMI and a lower aerobic capacity.

* ACTN3 – This is an endurance gene that may impact your performance and provide an advantage in sports requiring fast-twitch fibers.

*PPARA – A fat burning gene, this influences your body's ability to generate fuel from fat instead of carbs.

*COL5A1/COL1A1/MMP3 – These genes are associated with exercise-related tendon and ligament injuries.

*MYH7, MYBPC3, TNNT2, and TNNI3 – These are the genes that have been linked to the rare diseases called HCM, which is the most common cause of sudden cardiac death in athletes, and often misdiagnosed. There have been some high-profile athletes who have succumbed to this condition, but it most often occurs in high school athletes because symptoms typically start to surface during adulthood.

FUN FACT:

Research at UCLA demonstrates that exercise increases growth factors in the brain, making it easier for the brain to make new neuronal connections.[154]

THE FUTURE OF PROFESSIONAL SPORT

Malcolm Collins is an expert in sports genetics who studied the role genes played in tendon and ligament issues. He predicted that collagen genes could explain which athletes suffered injuries and which didn't. Dr. Stuart Kim at Stanford University has advanced the research involving genetics and sports injuries in professional athletes.

That research started in 2008, when Dr. Kim led a project to test 100 NFL linemen to search for a link between genetics and strength. What proved to be even more interesting to both him and the players was the link between genetics and injuries.

Injuries are one of the biggest threats to an athlete's career. Not only can a bad injury end a career, but it can impact performance and slow an athlete down. When it comes to some of the best athletes in the world, a fraction of a second can be the difference between a win and a loss, or first place and fourth.

Dr. Kim expanded his research, and after gaining access to large data sets of hundreds of thousands of people, he was better able to identify the genetic markers that determine different types of muscular skeletal injuries.[155] With that information, he created the company AxGen, which uses genetics to help athletes enhance training and prevent injury. Right now, they test to determine genetic susceptibility (normal, increased, or decreased) to ten specific sports injuries:

1. Thumb dislocation

2. Rotator cuff injury

3. MCL injury

4. Ankle sprain

5. Planter fasciitis

6. Stress fracture/bone mineral density

7. Achilles tendon injury

8. Concussion

9. ACL and PCL injury

10. Shoulder instability

Technology is rapidly evolving, and this list will grow along with it. Right now, the technology doesn't exist to reverse the genetic susceptibility, or eliminate injury altogether—injury will most likely always be a part of sports on every level. However, an athlete can benefit from this information by changing their training regimen accordingly to compensate for genetic weaknesses. The idea is to treat the mutation just as you would any other gene mutation. The approach taken comes down to what Dr. Kim refers to as the five P's:

- Predictive
- Personalized
- Preventative
- Participatory
- Professional athletes rely on percentage to win

The probability of ACL rupture has been traced to variants in the COL1A1 gene that impacts the amount of collagen the body produces. The less collagen your body produces, the higher the risk. Some people produce more, and are much less likely to suffer an ACL rupture because of it. If you know that you are susceptible to Achilles injury, you might consider altering your diet to help the tendons. You also want to strengthen the calves and leg muscles around the Achilles to protect the vulnerable tendon, while making sure your body isn't putting too much pressure on it.

One of the most common sports injuries is an ankle sprain, and there are genetic markers that can determine if you are more or less susceptible to that particular injury. When it comes to stress fracture, which can be a significant problem for endurance athletes, the biggest risk factor is bone density, and algorithms have been developed to predict bone density based on DNA.[156] If you are at risk, AxGen will lay out a plan to decrease your chance of injury that includes a bone scan, supplementation, stretching, low-impact training, cross training, biomechanical movement evaluation, and altering your footwear.

Before forming AxGen, Dr. Kim put this method to the test when applying it to the Stanford triathlon team, and they saw a significant decrease in these types of sports injuries. Genetics can also impact the way one absorbs and processes ibuprofen (used for inflammation) and caffeine (for energy), all of which can play a crucial factor in athletic performance.

It isn't only pro athletes who can benefit from this technology. AxGen offers these services to the public. It starts with a genomic analysis that is used to create personalized reports, exercise recommendations, and preventative measures all based on your genes. Right now, AxGen is one of the only companies that offer these services to the public, but more companies will follow as the technology advances.

FUN FACT:

Physical activity may help flush bacteria out of the lungs, reducing your chance of getting a cold and flu, which causing a change in white blood cells that serve as the body's immune system to help fight disease.[157]

TESTOSTERONE, FITNESS, AND AGING

Testosterone is an anabolic hormone and the primary sex hormone in men. It's responsible for the development of male sex organs, and influences mood, energy, and arousal. It also increases muscle mass, repairs damaged tissue, increases bone density, improves metabolism, reduces fat, increases energy, and acts as an anti-inflammatory agent. It's often called the youth hormone in men because testosterone levels increase rabidly during adolescence, peak when men are in their 20s, and begin to decline after the age of 30. Almost 40 percent of the men over 45 have low testosterone levels (less than 300 ng/dl)[158]

Women also produce testosterone, but in lower amounts. In women, testosterone levels are low during adolescence, but rise in middle age and during menopause. But just because you're a woman, that doesn't mean you can ignore testosterone. Too much testosterone can cause hair loss, acne, and infertility, and too little testosterone can lead to weak bones, loss of libido, and fertility problems, so it's important for both sexes to maintain healthy levels.

Other female hormones, like estrogen and progesterone, may act as a suppressor or promoter of inflammation. Scientists believe this may explain the need for a stronger response in the immune system of women when they are faced with foreign agents such as bacteria, viruses, parasites, and toxins. This may partially explain the reason for a higher incidence of autoimmune diseases in women when compared to men.

Symptoms of low testosterone include:

- Lack of energy
- Low libido
- Loss of lean body mass
- Loss of muscle and bone density
- Lack of motivation
- Fatigue

Low testosterone is associated with:

- Cardiovascular morbidity
- Metabolic syndromeDyslipidemia
- High blood pressure
- Stroke
- Atherosclerosis
- Osteoporosis
- Sarcopenia
- Depression
- Increased mortality risk

It becomes a continuous quest to build testosterone levels back up to increase energy and vigor. That's why you see so many clinics today addressing testosterone levels in men, and there is a whole slew of hormones, gels, creams, supplement pills, and injectables all geared toward the common goal of raising testosterone levels. In some cases, a doctor might even prescribe actual testosterone, but before you rush out to find a solution, it's important to first determine the cause.

There isn't just one cause. Balancing hormones involves complex systems, so it gets complicated. For instance, if someone comes into my clinic with the symptoms of low testosterone, I first do bloodwork to establish a baseline and see what those testosterone levels really are. Next, a functional medicine test takes the testosterone in your blood and follows it into the male hormonal pathway. Since everything leaves a marker, we can see what's going wrong and where. When we get the results from the functional medicine test, amongst other things, we learn the levels of cholesterol and DHEA, or dehydroepiandrosterone. DHEA is one of the most abundant steroid hormones and a precursor to testosterone.

This is where personalized medicine comes into play, because if someone has low levels of DHEA (and that person has converted their DHEA into testosterone), it means they have a DHEA problem and not a testosterone problem. In those cases, we can add a DHEA supplement. This can help people look and feel younger. I've tried it myself and it can work. However, you might also have the opposite problem in that you have a lot of DHEA, but it's not converting into testosterone, which means you have a conversion issue. Then, it doesn't matter how much DHEA you take, because your body won't convert it to active testosterone.

This is exactly why you can't just take supplements that you hear might have worked for someone else, because there are a lot of factors at play that might not make them as effective for you. It's why we do bloodwork, functional medicine tests, and then look at genomics because there are also certain genes responsible for processing testosterone, such ESR1. If someone has this gene mutation, and is also experiencing the symptoms of low testosterone, we work toward turning that gene off through nutrition, supplementation, and exercise, while building up the area that needs to be addressed.

Another possible cause could be your aromatase levels. Aromatase is an enzyme the body uses to regulate the conversion of testosterone to estradiol, which is a female sex hormone and basically a form of broken-down estrogen. Aromatase is found in fat cells, so when we gain fat, we increase are aromatase levels, and with it, estrogen. This is not ideal for men, so when you have low testosterone, you want to lower aromatase levels.[159]

Something else to look at are your SHBG1 and SHBG2 levels. These are sex hormone-binding globulin, which bind to testosterone and estradiol. The higher the SHBG in the blood, the more estrogen the body produces, and the lower the availability of free testosterone, which is the workhorse of our body. That's the anabolic portion of testosterone that repairs tissue and fuels our libido. As you can see, balancing hormones requires investigation, finesse, and also personalization.

What you can do today:

Oftentimes, lifestyle modifications are the best way to increase testosterone, and the natural approach doesn't have the potential side effects associated with certain medication. There are four things you can start doing immediately.

1. DIET: Foods like tuna, eggs, beef, beans, shellfish, and oysters can help raise testosterone levels along with foods high in zinc and vitamin D. Remove sugars, flours, and refined carbohydrates to reduce insulin sensitivity and ultimately lose fat.[160] If looking to decrease your aromatase levels, you can eat foods such as dietary fiber, flax seed, soy, grape seed extract, white button mushrooms, and green tea, which inhibit aromatase. Stinging nettle root is an herb that inhibits aromatase, as do quercetin, vitamin C, chrysin, and zinc.[161] Boosting your omega-3 levels can also help decrease aromatase. This can be a quick way to remove the interference in the production of testosterone.

2. GET MORE SLEEP: Sleep decreases cortisol, which can increase stress levels and interfere with the body's natural testosterone production.

3. LIMIT ALCOHOL CONSUMPTION: Alcohol also raises cortisol levels and interferes with the body's natural testosterone production.

4. EXERCISE: Arguably, the single-best thing you can do, starting today, to raise your testosterone levels is exercise. HIIT training and weight-lifting, specifically lower body exercises, such as squats and lunges, can raise those levels. Exercise also raises levels of HDL cholesterol, which is the healthy cholesterol. While unhealthy cholesterol becomes plaque that can harden and clog arteries, leading to high-blood pressure and cardio-vascular health issues, HDL cholesterol is used to make hormones, like testosterone. I've watched several patients of mine increase their healthy HDL levels 20 points (going from the 30s up to the 40s and 50s) through exercise alone.

It's a cycle. Testosterone increases your muscle development and ath-letic performance, and exercise can help raise your testosterone. No matter how you approach it, it all starts with and circles back to exercise. It doesn't matter what exercise you choose do at first—just get moving.

PART III

THE VARIABLES: PERSONALIZED GENOMICS

CHAPTER 8:

COMMON GENE MUTATIONS
AND HOW TO ADJUST

IT'S NO LONGER JUST A MATTER OF TAKING SUPPLEMENTS AND EATING WELL, but with genomics, you can take that to the next level by using nutrition and supplementation to compensate for the deficiencies resulting from genomic and epigenetic changes.

There are some genes that we know a lot about, and others we don't have as much information on. We may know what some of those genes do, some of the nutrients that can help them, and the pathways of the diseases associated with those genes, but there just hasn't been as much research conducted as there has been on other genes. But this will change as we acquire more and more data. And that is happening at a rapid pace. Just in the past few years, we know significantly more, and the reason is that more people have had their DNA analyzed and uploaded their data. With that data, we can spot trends and have quickly learned that some mutations are more common than others.

As a reminder:

Homozygous (+/+): You've inherited two mutated genes, one from each parent.

Homozygous (−/−): You've inherited two normal genes, one from each parent.

Heterozygous (+/−): You've inherited a mutated gene from one parent and a normal gene from another.

This is where epigenetics comes in. If you have (+/+) or two mutated genes from each parent, that mutation will most likely be expressed. Technically, the CRISPR-Cas9 procedure could cut out the bad gene and reconnect the strands of DNA back together to remove the chance of a possible mutation. That's why it's one of the greatest achievements in genetics, but we're probably 15 or 20 years away from that being applied to humans, and there are ethical concerns as well.

Unlike genetic changes, epigenetic changes are reversible and do not alter your DNA sequence, but they can change how your body reads that DNA sequence. For example, even if you have a (+/+) and that gene is expressed, we seek to provide support through nutrition, supplementation, and functional medicine. Even if you have a (−/−), that normal gene may be affected by epigenetic mechanisms that can influence the chromatin state, which in turn affects the expression of that gene. If it's total gene silencing, then the gene's action is killed, and no protein will be produced.

The genes we want to focus on are the heterozygous genes (+/−). This means you've inherited a normal gene from one parent and a mutated gene from another. That means that the gene might be expressed, or it might not. THIS IS THE PART OF GENETICS THAT YOU HAVE THE MOST SAY IN. If you don't have healthy eating habits, don't exercise regularly, or are exposed to environmental toxins, that gene will most likely be expressed. That is true for genes linked to everything from diabetes to cardiovascular disease, cancer, and even the longevity genes. Recently scientists discovered that the PCSK9 gene, which maintains the cholesterol levels in blood, and leads to extremely low cholesterol levels in those with a mutation. Pharmaceutical companies have developed drugs based on these findings.[162]

If you take care of yourself with proper nutrition, supplementation, and plenty of exercise, you can prevent those genes from being expressed. We're not talking about making any permanent changes, but we are trying to maximize the genome's efficiency based on epigenetic factors. Knowing this information can give you a fighting chance to prevent a mutated gene linked to certain conditions from being expressed.

Don't forget that mutations aren't always a bad thing. We are all mutants, and as we acquire more and more genetic data, we've noticed that some gene mutations are quite common. Here is a list of the most common mutations I've encountered consistently at my practice, what it means if you have that mutation, and what you can do about it.

COMT (catechol-O-methyltransferase)

"Breaking Down Dopamine"

I always associate this gene with conditions like OCD, ADHD, a tendency toward perfectionism, other mental disorders, and also various eating disorders.

David, a patient of mine with this mutation, had such a severe case of OCD that he would frequently go out to his garage and clean the gravel between the stones on the floor with a toothbrush. When that didn't work, he'd use a toothpick. In this case, we did a full genomic analysis, and a brain neurotransmitter functional medicine test to determine the proper supplementation, and I recommended him for behavioral therapy.

Not everyone will have this reaction. I personally have this gene mutation, which drives me toward tendencies of perfection, and I don't always view that as a negative trait. It's part of what led to my fascination with this very topic.

The Science

If you have a COMT mutation, your brain neurotransmitters will likely be off. Serotonin, dopamine, and norepinephrine are all neurotransmitters that play a role in attention span, language, and reward-seeking behavior. It creates pleasurable feelings and reinforces the behaviors that lead to those feelings. Dopamine levels play a role in conditions like Parkinson's disease. This mutation can also impact estrogen, which can translate to being more sensitive to pain. Methyl B12 may be tolerated better by those who are (−/−) as compared to those who are (+/+) or (+/−).

The Nutrition

With this mutation, you want to eat more cruciferous vegetables, such as cabbage, broccoli, cauliflower, Brussels sprouts, and flaxseed to support estrogen metabolism.

The Supplements

- Adenosyl/Hydroxy B12 from Pure Encapsulation (liquid preferred).
- L-theanine from Vital Nutrients.

Many of my patients with this mutation found almost immediate relief from the L-theanine. We started with one capsule per day at first, but when he felt that wasn't strong enough, we upped that to two, and it gave him a tremendous amount of relief. His wife noticed a difference in his behavior, and felt that he was calmer, demonstrated fewer OCD tendencies, and his coping mechanisms improved. It's important to note that L-theanine can provide relief for various eating disorders, and I have witnessed this quite a bit in my own practice.

FUN FACT:

The COMT gene goes far in determining our personalities, since the enzyme the gene codes for breaks down neurotransmitters in the brain's frontal lobe, which is responsible for things like short-term memory, our planning abilities, behavioral inhibitions, and our reaction to stress.[163]

VDR

"The Vitamin D Receptor"

We've all been told how being out in the sun is an excellent source of vitamin D, and that's true, but don't assume that you can get all your necessary allotment of vitamin D only from the sun. I have many patients from the beach cities in Southern California who are out in the sun all of the time, yet their vitamin D levels are still below normal. The reason is that they have this mutation, and their bodies can't process it, whether it's internally or externally.

It used to be expensive to get your vitamin D levels checked, but now it's part of standard bloodwork as most family practitioners almost always add it to their panel. The normal range for vitamin D is 30 to 50 ng/mL,[164] though I believe that 60 to 80 ng/mL is the preferred range for optimal function. When your levels are low, you may experience fatigue, aches, thyroid issues, hormonal imbalance, adrenal gland exhaustion, and even cancer.[165] Low vitamin D is an underlying condition in many diseases, which is why it's been making a lot of headlines lately for the role it plays in our overall health.

The Science

Despite the name, vitamin D isn't a vitamin, but a hormone produced in the skin and converted by the liver and kidneys. It supports function in the brain, muscles, and immune system. It's also required for the intestinal absorption of dietary calcium and phosphorus, which aids in bone and teeth formation. That's why vitamin D deficiency can result in the softening of bones: osteoporosis in adults and rickets in children. It also aids in pancreas function by keeping blood sugar in a healthy range.[166]

The Nutrition

Good sources of vitamin D are mushrooms, fish, milk, and other dairy products. Fish like tuna, salmon, swordfish, herring, sardines, and even cod liver oil are all good sources of vitamin D. However, you want to be careful when consuming too much tuna and swordfish, because they can increase your mercury levels.

The Supplements

- Vitamin D3 with K2 from Pure Encapsulations (liquid preferred).
- Vitamin D3 + K from Metagenics.
- Liposomal Vitamin D3 – Manna.
- Vitamin K2-7 + D3 from Vital Nutrients

The Liposomal supplements tend to be more expensive. They have a fatty substance that (like MCT) that helps the vitamins and nutrients get through the cell membrane and into the cell. Liposomal helps you get more out of the supplements.

Some patients with this mutation who were deficient in vitamin D were placed on a regimen of 10,000 IU vitamin D3 supplement once a week, and it still wasn't enough to raise the level of vitamin D in their blood to 30. They had to take a vitamin D3 supplement every day. When we tested them again after three months, their levels went up, and their symptoms disappeared. With vitamin D, it's all about the dose and the frequency. Results also depend on the person, but I've noticed that patients typically experience a difference in 30 days. Just keep in mind that the bioavailability can be reduced by certain medications.

Early in the pandemic of 2020, doctors learned that elderly patients who had previously taken vitamin D3 supplements were more likely to survive COVID-19, while those with a deficiency in vitamin D3 experienced more severe symptoms.[167]

Warning!

If supplementing with vitamin D, it's important to note that it's a fat-soluble vitamin, which means that you CAN take too much and overload your system over time. Fat-soluble vitamins (like vitamins A, E, K, and CoQ10) require fat to be broken down, and can cause toxins to build up in your system, but they are absorbed better when taken with fat.[168] Dosage is important, and depending on your genes, taking 10,000 IU at one time, though beneficial in certain instances, might be too much. This is unlike a water-soluble vitamin, such as vitamin C. On average, you can take up to

3,500 milligrams of vitamin C, and your body won't have any issue absorbing it. If you do end up taking too much vitamin C, the side effects are minimal, but the best way to usually tell if you're taking too much is if you have watery stools, nausea, loss of appetite, fatigue, and diarrhea.

FUN FACT:

Vitamin D is the only vitamin in your body that actually makes itself, which is why it's considered more of a hormone.[169]

MAOA (MONOAMINE OXIDASE A)

"Breaks Down Serotonin"

This mutation goes hand-in-hand with COMT and is one of the main culprits of OCD. Like dopamine, serotonin is another neurotransmitter involved with mood regulation, and is also associated with depression, aggression, and anxiety, which is why it's often called the "warrior gene." This mutation is common in those with anorexia and other eating disorders. When I have a patient with both a COMT and an MAOA mutation, it usually results in more severe symptoms.

The Science

The MAOA gene codes for the enzyme monoamine oxidase, which breaks down neurotransmitters such as noradrenaline, adrenaline, serotonin, and dopamine, which is how it can regulate mood. MAOA is located on the X chromosome, so women can be heterozygous or homozygous. Men only have one X chromosome and are therefore hemizygous.[170] Since the X chromosome in males can only come from the mother, the father's MAOA mutations (or lack thereof) do not play a role in their son's MAOA status. For females, since one X chromosome is inherited from each parent, the genetics tend to reflect the MAOA status of both parents.[171]

Recommended Supplementation

- L-theanine from Vital Nutrients.
- 5HTP by Pure Encapsulations.

Nutrition and supplementation won't cure anxiety, depression, OCD, or an eating disorder, but I have seen the severity of many of my patients' symptoms decrease with the proper supplementation. That allows them to function better in relationships and feel better. Some discover that the things that used to trigger their episodes are less impactful, or that they are better able to sit with those uncomfortable feelings with more ease.

MTHFR (METHYLENETETRAHYDROFOLATE REDUCTASE)
"The Methylation Gene"

This is a big one! There are eight core genes involved in methylation, but MTHFR is the main one, and if you have this mutation, you will have issues with methylation. As you know by now, methylation is life, and some significant symptoms and conditions can occur from being over- or under-methylated. It can be associated with increased risk of cardiovascular disease, depression, schizophrenia, birth defects, Down syndrome, psoriasis, diabetes, Parkinson's disease, and various cancers.

The Science

The methylation pathway starts with MTHFR, and it has one job: to turn folic acid into folate. Folic acid is a man-made nutrient that we get from processed foods that are fortified with B vitamins.[172] This is so common, and in my experience, 60 to 80 percent of my patients have this gene mutation, which means they don't benefit from the B vitamin cycle working optimally.

Several mutations in the MTHFR gene have been well characterized as increasing the risk of heart disease and cancer and may play a role in the level of serotonin and dopamine. There are a lot of pathways that are dependent on MTHFR, so it's an extremely important gene.

Recommended Nutrition

When you have this mutation, it's best to avoid foods with folic acid, such as broccoli, Brussels sprouts, and leafy green vegetables. However, not all experts agree that folic acid is an issue if you have this mutation. There is a current debate about this, but this just goes to show how there is still a lot we don't yet know when it comes to our genes.

Recommended Supplementation

- Adenosyl/Hydroxy B12
  ▷ Pure Encapsulations (Liquid preferred).
  ▷ Holistic Health.
- 5-MTHF
  ▷ Metagenics – Included in the "Wellness Essentials" multivitamin.
  ▷ Vital Nutrients. Included in the "Multi–Nutrients," multivitamin.
  ▷ Thorne 5-MTHF1

This gene converts folic acid to methyl folate (5MTHF or B9) using B12. This gene relies heavily on B12 to function well, so supplementation and nutrition are the best way to provide immediate support, along with exercise, maintaining a low-stress level, and removing toxins. If the gene is homozygous (+/+), there is nothing you can do to change that, but you can reinforce the pathway. The B12 does a lot of work for the methylation cycle, so this supplement can help so many different ailments because life does not exist without proper methylation.

FUN FACT:

Every single cell and tissue in your body experiences methylation.[173]

MTR/MTRR (METHIONINE SYNTHASE/METHIONINE SYNTHASE REDUCTASE)

"The B12 Gene"

These gene mutations are very similar to the MTHFR gene, as they also aid in methylation. Most symptoms can be improved significantly by supplementing with B12.

The Science

The MTR gene uses methyl folate and methylcobalamin (B12) to turn homocysteine into methionine. The MTRR gene provides instructions for making an enzyme called methionine synthase, which helps process amino acids.[174] These genes use B12 to convert homocysteine to methionine. High levels of homocysteine have been linked to conditions such as heart disease and Alzheimer's disease. When you have this mutation, B12 is used at a much faster rate, which is why supplementation is so important.

Recommended Nutrition

Just like with the MTHFR mutation, you want to add more folate to your diet in the form of avocados, leafy green vegetables, and lentils.

Recommended Supplementation

- Adenosyl/Hydroxy B12
  - ▷ Pure Encapsulations (liquid preferred).
  - ▷ Holistic Health.
- 5MTHF
  - ▷ As part of "Wellness Essentials" from Metagenics.
  - ▷ As part of Vital Nutrients called "Multi – Nutrients," from Vital Nutrients.
  - ▷ Thorne has a single-nutrient 5-MTHF 1.

CBS (cystathionine-beta synthase)

"Everything Sulfur Related"

When you eat foods high in sulfur, you need the enzyme to help you break that down, so if someone has the CBS mutation, you may have trouble breaking down foods high in sulfur. And a lot of foods are high in sulfur, such as leafy green vegetables like cabbage, broccoli, and kale.

This is where it becomes personalized medicine, because many experts mean well when they say, "Eat more kale! Kale is great!" But if you have the CBS mutation, you won't be able to break down kale as well, so if you eat too much kale, you would actually be overwhelming your system with sulfur. You also want to be careful of dried fruits and nuts and want to find brands without sulfur. Too much sulfur can create a buildup of ammonia, leading to gout and other kidney issues.[175] Those with a CBS mutation may experience headaches, brain fog, and a lack of concentration.

The Science

This enzyme breaks down homocysteine to sulfur end-products. Mutations can decrease the support for the rest of the methylation pathway, including B12, to address the MTR and MTRR mutations, while producing excess ammonia and sulfites. The CBS gene requires B6 and iron, and since CBS also aids in the production of glutathione, someone with this mutation can have a problem with toxins building up in their system. That's why detoxification is so important at the start because it can help clear your pathways, so the body functions properly and can process nutrients and supplements.

Recommended Nutrition

If you have this mutation, you want to avoid foods with sulfur, such as garlic, onions, and vegetables like broccoli, cauliflower, and kale in favor of meats, cereals, peas, and beans.

Recommended Supplementation

- Molybdenum Glycinate
  ▷ Thorne.
  ▷ Pure Encapsulations, as part of "Trace Nutrients."

It's beneficial to avoid foods with sulfur when you have this mutation, but if you decide to start supplementing (in this case with molybdenum), your body should be able to break down sulfur much better, so you can slowly reintroduce those foods back into your diet. I've personally seen this supplement significantly help patients.

BHMT (betaine homocysteine methyltransferase)

"The Backup for the Liver and Kidneys"

You can also consider the BHMT gene a backup system for methylation as well. If someone has methylation issues, the BHMT gene will kick in. Consider it like a Plan B or a spare tire. You never want this gene to be your driving force, because eventually it will break down. Just keep in mind that if you have both an MTHFR mutation and a BHMT mutation, that means it will require more work and patience. Even though they are similar, BHMT is a different enzyme than MTHFR and that requires a different nutrition and supplement regimen. In my experience, if you have both mutations, it's advised to work on correcting the MTHFR mutation first.

The Science

This gene makes methionine from choline and TMG, and is essentially the shortcut through the methylation cycle, helping to convert homocysteine to methionine. The gene activity can be affected by stress and cortisol levels, so it may play a role in ADD and ADHD by affecting norepinephrine levels. Those with this mutation may benefit from additional shortcut support. The cofactor in BHMT is choline, and not B2 like it is in MTRR, so it requires choline or betaine to function better.

Recommended Nutrition

Since this gene helps to convert homocysteine to methionine, the nutrition is similar to that of an MTHFR and MTR mutation in that you want to avoid foods with folic acid.

Recommended Supplementation

- For BHMT2:
  - ▷ Phosphatidylserine (PSC) as a single nutrient from Orthomolecular Products.

- For BHMT8:
  - ▷ Adenosyl/Hydroxy B12.
    - · Pure Encapsulations (liquid preferred).
    - · Holistic Health.

NAT 1 AND NAT 2

These are great antioxidant markers that detoxify many environmental toxins like smoke and exhaust. When I think of NAT1 and NAT2, I think of cellular oxidation, mitochondria, and the energy that drives cell function. These genes play a significant role in helping the liver detox and are part of the Cytochrome P450 pathway. So when you have these mutations, it can lead to fatigue, and since it's also involved in removing toxins, it can result in skin issues like acne and eczema. Mutations may also result in rapid acetylation that comes with a risk of lung, colon, bladder, and head and neck cancer. [176]

The Science

Both NAT1 and NAT2 are used in the acetylation of numerous environmental toxins, so a mutation in these genes can lead to the inability to properly clear toxins, which increases the risk of lung, colon, breast, bladder, and head and neck cancer. Urinary cancer appears to have the most consistent association with slow acetylation.

Recommended Supplementation

- Antioxidants
  - ▷ Indigo Greens from Orthomolecular Products.
  - ▷ Deeper Greens from Metagenics.
- Fish oil
  - ▷ Metagenics.
  - ▷ Nordic Naturals.
- Liposomal glutathione from Pure Encapsulations
  ACAT1

The ACAT1 gene is responsible for cellular energy production within the mitochondria, which produces energy in the form of ATP (adenosine triphosphate) that all of our cells, organs, and systems depend on. It provides instructions for making the enzyme that helps to break down proteins by processing isoleucine, and fats by processing ketones. It also indirectly impacts the methylation cycle by depleting B12, so it's in the same category as MTHFR and MTRR and will require similar nutrition and supplementation.

Recommended Supplementation

- ResveraCel from Thorne.
- Mitochondria ATP from Pure Encapsulations.
- Mitovive from Metagenics.
- Mitocore from Orthomolecular Products.
- COq10 ST 100 from Metagenics.
- Acetyl L— Carnitine from Vital Nutrients.

AHCY

AHCY converts adenosyl homocysteine (SAH) to adenosine and homocysteine. It's similar to a CBS mutation and can often benefit from similar treatment. It's a part of the methylation pathway, and its primary function is to produce S-adenosylmethionine (SAMe), a major methyl donor. A deficiency in SAMe has been linked to depression.

Recommended Supplementation

- SAMe as a single nutrient from Orthomolecular Products.

SUOX

Not everyone tests for this gene, but it is an important one. The SUOX gene encodes for a protein called sulfite oxidase. It allows sulfur to be stored as glutathione. Think of it as your body's garbage disposal. It picks up the byproducts of the methylation cycle, like sulfites, and removes them from our system. It keeps things moving, so none of those byproducts can go back into circulation and cause more issues. The effects and treatment are very similar to that of a CBS mutation.

Recommended Supplementation

- Molybdenum Glycinate.
  - ▷ Thorne.

- As part of "Trace Minerals"
  - ▷ Pure Encapsulations.

MAT

Similar to the SUOX, the MAT gene controls the production of SAMe. It also aids in DNA methylation, gene expression, and helps to remove sulfur from the body while balancing homocysteine levels.

Recommended Supplementation

- SAMe – As a single nutrient from Orthomolecular Products.
- SAMe as a single nutrient from Pure Encapsulations.

GSTM1 AND GSTT1

Glutathione S-Transferase, specifically GSTM1 and GSTT1, may not be a common gene mutation, but they are important ones and possibly lethal. These genes are involved in the detoxification of potentially carcinogenic agents, and if you have these mutations, you are more susceptible to certain cancers.[177] I've seen this first-hand. My patients with these mutations either have cancer or an immediate history of cancer in their families—some with extremely rare forms of cancer. What happens is that your body doesn't produce enough glutathione, a major antioxidant that fights free radicals and protects cells from toxins. Glutathione S-Transferase is a family of 13 proteins located in different organs. Different isoforms (a set of highly similar proteins that originate from a single gene or gene family) are located in the liver, kidney, pancreas, ovaries, small intestine, brain, and heart, so when mutated, those areas are more likely to be affected. That's why a person with this mutation should be taking a glutathione supplement for the rest of their lives.

Recommended Supplementation

- Liposomal glutathione from Pure Encapsulations.
- Liposomal glutathione from Manna.
- NAC 600 mg from Vital Nutrients.
- NAD(H) from Ecological formulas.
- Basis from Elysium

Hopefully, you're beginning to see the pattern to remove the irritant through detox, replace the deficiency with supplementation and nutrition to repair the gene, thus restoring its function. The detox is crucial, because if there is toxicity (metal, non-metal, or environmental) and you don't remove it, you can do everything else right and live a healthy life, but toxicity will continue to affect your DNA, and subsequently your cells, tissues, organs, organ systems, and ultimately your function as a human being.

ADDITIONAL MUTATIONS

- GPx1P1
  - ▷ What it does: Reduces capacity to detoxify hydrogen peroxide.
  - ▷ What to do: If (+/+) or (−/+), try eating a diet rich in fruits and cruciferous vegetables, and supplement with antioxidants.
- GSTP1
  - ▷ What it does: Reduces the ability to conjugate some toxins with glutathione.
  - ▷ What to do: If (+/+) or (−/+), try eating a diet rich in fruits and cruciferous vegetables, and supplement to support detoxification.
- NQO1
  - ▷ What it does: It's associated with reduced enzyme activity.
  - ▷ What to do: If (+/+) or (−/+), limit your exposure to tobacco smoke, get regular exercise, and eat a diet rich in cruciferous vegetables.
- SOD2
  - ▷ What it does: Alters the distribution of the SOD2 enzyme, which may compromise antioxidant defenses.
  - ▷ What to do: If (+/+) or (−/+), eat a diet high in cruciferous vegetables and foods rich in lycopene and other antioxidants. You want to support breast and prostate health if you have this mutation.
- FUT2

- ▷ What it does: There is a modified risk of low B12 status and the potential for lower-intestinal microbial diversity.
- ▷ What to do: If (+/+), include yogurt, kefir, and fermented foods in your diet. If (−/+) or (−/−), supplement with B12.

- TCN2
  - ▷ What it does: This mutation is associated with lower levels of bioavailable B12.
  - ▷ What to do: If (+/+) or (−/+), supplement with B12.

- BCM01 (A379V, R2672)
  - ▷ What it does: This reduces your ability to convert dietary beta-carotene to active vitamin A.
  - ▷ What to do: If (+/+) or (−/+), make sure you get enough vitamin A from supplements or foods like organ meats, eggs, cod liver oil, and dairy products.

- GC
  - ▷ What it does: This may limit your ability to deliver vitamin D3 to cells.
  - ▷ What to do: If (+/+) or (−/−), a vitamin D supplement is recommended.

- SLC20A8
  - ▷ What it does: This may impact your body's levels of zinc.
  - ▷ What to do: If (+/+) or (−/+), make sure you get enough zinc.

- SLC23A1
  - ▷ What it does: This is associated with low levels of vitamin C.
  - ▷ What to do: If (+/+), make sure you get enough vitamin C through citrus fruits, berries, or supplementation.

CHAPTER 9:

LONGEVITY AND LIVING TO 100

AGING IS INEVITABLE. AS ALL LIVING ORGANISMS AGE, THERE IS A DECLINE in the function of organs and systems, leading to an increase in oxidative stress, tissue deterioration, and cell death. There is nothing that we as humans can do to stop the aging process, but our genes hold the secret for how to delay it.

In 2003, Dan Buettner set off on a series of National Geographic expeditions to discover the secrets of longevity in so-called "longevity hotspots" where people consistently lived to be 100. Sardinia, Italy; Okinawa, Japan; Loma Linda, California; Nicoya Peninsula, Costa Rica; and Icaria, Greece became known as the "blue zones." Buettner spoke about his findings and also published a book called *The Blue Zones*.[178] There was no one link to longevity, but he did find some core commonalities. Diet, exercise, stress, lifestyle, community, and a sense of belonging all played a role in the longevity of the Blue Zone people, but for many centenarians around the globe, their longevity is linked more directly to genetics.

FUN FACT:

Global life expectancy has risen more than seven years since 1990, equivalent to a year gained every three-and-a-half years.[179]

IT'S ALL ABOUT THE TELOMERES

We can't talk about the aging process and longevity without discussing telomeres, because they play a vital role in cellular health and longevity. This word derives from the Greek words "telo" meaning "end" and "mere" meaning "part," but it pertains to the cells in the biological context.[180] We've learned a lot about telomeres in recent years. The 2009 Nobel Prize in Medicine or Physiology was awarded to Elizabeth H. Blackburn, Carol W. Greider, and Jack W. Szostak for discoveries related to telomeres.[181]

Telomeres are located at the end of the chromosomes and are commonly compared to the plastic ends of a shoelace that provide protection and stability, and just like those protective caps on shoelaces, these telomeres keep your DNA from fraying and breaking down. Telomeres have repetitive DNA sequences comprised of six nucleotides (TTGGGG) at the end of each chromosome. They have two primary functions:

1. They protect the cell against chromosomal fusions.
2. They are used as buffers when there is a replication issue.

Telomeres don't have any genes, so they don't produce or code for any proteins. But without telomeres, the cell would try to repair what looks like a break in the DNA, and that would result in harmful chromosomal fusions and genetic instability.[182]

Cells die every day and are replicated based on our original DNA template. Whenever the cell divides, it becomes a new cell. However, when our DNA is replicated, it's not replicated all the way to the end, so we lose a small portion of these telomeres after every replication. No genetic information is lost because telomeres do not contain any genes. But as this occurs throughout our lifetime, the telomeres shorten to the point where they can no longer divide or replicate.

Newborns have telomeres ranging from 8,000 to 13,000 base pairs, with that number decreasing between 20 and 40 each year. By the age of 40, you might have lost 1,600 base pairs of the telomeres on each chromosome, and each time a cell divides, between 25 and 200 base pairs are lost due to either the end replication problem, or oxidate stress, which can be affected by lifestyle and diet.[183] If we're talking about a skin cell, that means it will replicate and divide until it can no longer create new cells. At that point, the skin starts to age. So, telomeres function almost as a cell-aging clock.

On average, cells can divide between 40 and 60 times before they reach the Hayflick limit, which is the number of times a cell will divide before it deteriorates and eventually stops dividing. That directly corresponds with the length of the telomeres on a given chromosome. Long story short, the longer the telomeres, the better the cellular performance.

Telomere length varies across human tissue types, but when they get too short, the cells enter crisis, which is when functional telomeres are lost. Chromosomal fusions and genomic instability occur, followed by widespread cell death. Decreased telomere length has been associated with many diseases, including atherosclerosis, osteoarthritis, osteoporosis, vascular dementia, pulmonary fibrosis, major depressive disorders, coronary artery disease, infertility, type 2 diabetes, and some cancers.[184] Some lifestyle behaviors like smoking, stress, and lack of exercise have been shown to shorten telomeres. Studies have also shown that those who have been subject to violence have shorter telomeres. Lack of sleep, obesity, excessive alcohol consumption, and drug addiction have all been associated with causing the telomeres to shorten. On the other hand, a healthy lifestyle that involves proper diet, exercise, meditation, and omega-3 fish oils has been shown to be effective in influencing telomere length.[185]

Cells can avoid death by stabilizing telomere length and expressing the enzyme telomerase, which lengthens telomeres and allows cells to maintain their length by becoming immortal. Telomerase is highly expressed in cancer cells, which essentially become immortal, but in non-pathological conditions, telomerase is expressed in early stages of embryo development and in some adult stem cell compartments. Interestingly enough, germ cells (sperm and egg) also express the telomerase enzyme.

I recommend initially measuring the length of your telomeres every six months for two years, and then once you can make positive lifestyle changes, have this done as part of your physical exam once a year. This can be done through the following trusted sources.

- SpectraCell Laboratories – Telomere Testing.
- RepeatDX – Telomere Testing for healthcare professionals.
- TeloYears – Genetic Testing.
- Life Length – Telomere Length and Biological Age Testing.

When the telomeres are too short, our DNA is at risk, and so cell division is halted to protect our DNA and chromosomes. This is called "senescence." It's when a healthy and vibrant cell that continues to divide becomes a non-dividing cell, which remains metabolically active and alive, but in a much different way: it looks different, behaves different, expresses different genes, and responds to the surrounding cells in a different way. Think of it like a zombie cell. The Hayflick limit is the natural way cells reach senescence. Senescence can also be a byproduct of DNA damage due to inflammation, infection, mutation, oxidative stress, and the exposome.

Senescent cells stop dividing as a way to prevent DNA damage and the cells from becoming cancerous. However, it's also a double-edged sword. On the one hand, it protects us from cancer by not allowing cell division of damaged DNA; but on the other hand, as we naturally age and have more senescent cells, our body can't repair itself as well as it once did. Mice may have longer telomeres than humans, but since mice and jellyfish have the same six nucleotide telomere sequence as humans, studies are being conducted to extend the lifespan by increase telomerase activity without promoting cancer. In one study, telomerase-treated mice, both at one year and at two years of age, had an increase in median lifespan of 24 and 13 percent, respectively.[186]

Cellular senescence impairs cell function and predisposes tissues, organs, and organ systems to disease and aging. Critically short telomeres, oxidative stress, environmental toxins, exposome, and the activation of cancer-driven genes known as oncogenes can all trigger cellular senescence. There are two ways to remove and replace senescent cells, the first being apoptosis, and the second being the availability of stem cell reserves. However, the accumulation of senescent cells can deplete stem cell reserves and impair their function.

This can degrade and destroy proteins while also causing inflammation. The overstimulation of senescent cells can decrease nitric oxide, which can lead to atherosclerosis, hypertension, hypercholesterolemia, diabetes mellitus, congestive heart failure, thrombosis and stroke, which have all been linked to abnormalities in nitric oxide signaling.[187] Accumulation of cellular senescence has been linked to diet-induced diabetes, liver and kidney issues, and enlarged prostate associated with benign prostate hypertrophy (BPH). Some studies have suggested that low back pain that is a result of intervertebral disc degeneration may also be due to cellular senescence.

When it comes to treatment for senescence, there are three primary methods.

1. Prevention: Simply put, take care of yourself, and monitor your telomere health with regular testing. You want to maintain cellular integrity and the DNA damage repair systems like the immune system and the P53 pathway. Not to sound like a broken record, but it's just another reason to detox regularly and make sure you supplement properly.
2. Removal: This is the body's system of recycling and removing cellular debris, which is also known as autophagy. The detox can help aid this

recycling and removal process, while also boosting immunity. It's just another reason why the detox is so important; it helps to minimize the exposure to harmful toxins and the need for more senescence.

3. Replacement: After the removal of senescence cells, replacement would include the addition of stem cells into the tissue.

FUN FACT:

Research teams determined that the lifespan of other species can be increased by genetic interventions, certain proteins, or dietary changes. In recent years, aging in mice could be reversed with telomerase, and similar experiments were conducted successfully with human cells.[188]

THE MAIN LONGEVITY GENES

A Danish twin study determined that how long a person lives is 20 percent genetic and 80 percent lifestyle,[189] but with the proper diet, exercise, and healthy lifestyle choices, the following genes can become significant assets, if you are one of the fortunate few to have them.

1. FOXO3

This is the primary longevity gene and the one we know the most about. If you have inherited both (+/+), you can live a very long life as long as you protect them. Of course, this doesn't mean you're invincible. Some unexpected outside factors and behaviors can impact your lifespan, but if you take care of yourself, from a genetics standpoint, you have the potential to make it to 100. Many centenarians studied have both copies of the FOXO3 gene, but even if you only have one copy of the gene, it can still have a major impact on your longevity. So, in the case of FOXO3, having only one of the genes is significantly better than having none. It's a blessing to preserve it.

Given what we're learning about genomics, we're just scratching the surface, so the possibilities are endless.

2. SIRT1 & SIRT6

Researchers at the University of Rochester released a study published in the journal *Cell*, linking SIRT6 to longevity because of its role in organizing proteins and recruiting enzymes that repair broken DNA.[190]

Haim Cohen, PhD., director of the Sagol Healthy Human Longevity Center at Bar-Ilan University, led an international study that determined that SIRT6 controls the rate of healthy aging in mice, and allowed them to better overcome age-related diseases, such as cancer and blood disorders. The mice who expressed high levels of SIRT6 had their life expectancy increase by an average of 30 percent. They found that the gene activates a physical response similar to intermittent fasting and diets that have been shown to increase longevity.[191]

These genes are more common among the Asian population, and both are responsible for how the DNA repairs itself and the aging of the brain, so it's been linked to longer lifespans. Not everyone has the SIRT1 and SIRT6 enzyme, but research has shown that certain nutrients, such as reservatrol (RSV), which is a compound found in the skin of red grapes, can mimic the enzyme activity of SIRT1 and SIRT6. It was found to increase the lifespan in yeast, worms, flies and fish, while in humans it was found to delay replicative aging by mobilization of antioxidant and DNA repair mechanisms.[192] This is just another way that you can utilize diet and lifestyle changes to improve longevity.

It's extremely rare, but I have treated siblings who have the best versions of both of the longevity genes: SIRT1 and FOXO3. I've worked with the Miller family for years. They ask questions, are attentive, and want to learn. They are the epitome of healthy lifestyle and living. They also have genetics working in their favor. Their father is from the United States and part English and French, while their mother is Cambodian and 15 percent Vietnamese. He has the best version of the FOXO3 gene, and she has the best version of the SIRT1 gene, and their two kids have inherited both genes. It's the best of both worlds, and it's the only time I've personally ever seen that. Most people typically either have one or the other—or neither. We've done genomic testing for each of those two children, so we know what they are predisposed to, but with proper diet and a healthy lifestyle, they have the genetic benefit of longevity.

THE GUARDIAN OF THE GENOME

P53 is an intriguing and complex pathway that includes more than 67 genes. The human p53 gene is located on the seventeenth chromosome, and it gets its name from its molecular mass—it is in the 53 kilodalton fraction of cell proteins. It's often referred to as the guardian of the genome, because it makes a protein in the nucleus of the cell that helps to control cell division and cell death. P53 promotes cellular stability and helps the cell function normally by reducing potential harmful mutations to the cells and their daughter cells during cell division. Once the p53 mechanism is activated, the cell is impacted three ways:

1. DNA repair and back to normal cellular function.

2. Cell growth arrest, which halts the progression of the cell cycle and prevents the replication of damaged DNA.

3. Programmed cell death or apoptosis.

If the damage done to the cell is repairable, the p53 will fix it. But if the cellular damage is beyond repair, the p53 system will program scheduled cell death to avoid errors in the cell reproduction process, which may result in faulty cellular DNA instructions and the production of the wrong protein, or a malfunction of existing proteins.

P53 is always active within cells. In healthy cells, the level of p53 protein is low, but the pathway is a cellular sensor, or an indicator of cellular distress, that becomes activated due to DNA damage, chemicals, radiation, viruses, hypoxia (a decrease in cellular oxygen levels), nutrient deprivation, oncogene expression (the presence of tumor and/or cancer cells), exposome, and epigenetics. Ribosomal stress can also activate the pathway, and since ribosomes are the workhorse of the cell and their main function is to convert DNA into proteins, this can impact the very building blocks of life.

These factors can all increase that level of activity due to unrepairable DNA damage. If there is too much p53 activity, cells can shut down and become senescent, which accelerates chronic inflammation, abnormal tissue breakdown, and tissue degradation.[193] New research has shown that cellular damage over time negatively impacts health and results in aging. Senescent cells can impair tissue function, so removing them can delay the aging process.[194] In fact, healthy p53 protein has been shown to suppress the DNA damage to the telomeres, which directly impacts longevity. However, if there is too little activity, precancerous cells might survive and form a tumor. If the p53 gene is damaged, tumor suppression is significantly reduced, which is why the p53 protein sits at the intersection of cancer and aging. The p53 has been shown to be mutated in more than 53 types of cancer, and 50 percent of all human tumors contain p53 mutations.[195] And those who inherit only one copy of p53 are more likely to develop tumors in early adulthood.[196]

Those who were physically inactive and who consumed a Western-style diet (fast food, trans-fatty acids, etc.) were more likely to have a p53 mutation.[197] That's why a low-carbohydrate or Mediterranean diet is recommended to maintain optimal p53 health. However, you can also naturally stimulate p53 activity through:

- Cruciferous vegetables such as broccoli, Brussels sprouts, cabbage, cauliflower, collard greens, arugula, and Bok choy.
- Food high in polyphenols such as red wine, black and green tea, soy, vegetables, nuts, beans, non-berry fruits, berries, cocoa powder, dark chocolate, and cloves.
- Teas and coffees.
- Vitamin C.
- Vitamin D.

- Food high in selenium like pork, beef, turkey, chicken, fish, shell-fish, and eggs.

- Herbs such as curcumin, scutellaria baicalensis, gleditsia sinen-sis thorns, kanglaite, thymoquinone (black seed oil), the honokiol, resveratrol, and baicalin.[198]

At the end of the day, our choices can either help or hurt our body's systems. This includes the way we think and live, and what we eat. This is another reason why I recommend the detox twice a year (the 10-day and 28-day) as part of a healthy lifestyle. It will help to protect the integrity of the cells and the cell membranes that house our DNA, and can limit the prolonged intense activation of the p53 genomic cascade. If we respect our genome, then the guardian of the genome will continue to protect us.

OTHER LONGEVITY GENES AND PATHWAYS

The aging process and longevity are complicated because one gene can activate other genes and pathways, but there is a distinct pattern. Much of anti-aging is driven by preventing senescence, or cell death. Telomeres play an important role in that. FOXO3, SIRT1, SIRT6, MTor, Daf-16, Daf-2, and IGF-1 are all genomic longevity genes and pathways that work together. Improving the health of each of these genes and their respective pathways plays a role and contributes a little more to your overall longevity. These genes also regulate chronic conditions. If you take care of your genome, and ensure the health of these longevity genes, you not only have the potential to live longer, but you're also increasing your health, so you can live better. Here are some of the more significant genes and pathways associated with aging and longevity:

- Cytochrome P450 – We spoke about cytochrome P450 during the detox section, but it's also relevant to longevity because there are 18 mammalian cytochrome P450 families, which encode for 57 genes. These genes are crucial to essential life processes. They metabo-lize drugs and other environmental chemicals, so defects can lead to serious conditions and diseases, such as glaucoma, vitamin D deficiency, hypertension, and coronary artery disease.[199] That makes this family of genes a significant part of the anti-aging process, which is why I recommend the detox. Get this family of genes to work for you, and it can become the equivalent of a longevity gene.

- IGF-1 – This system is complex, but simply put, it impacts the body's production of insulin and plays an essential role in the development of age-related diseases, such as cancer, dementia, cardiovascular disease, and metabolic diseases.[200] This is a pathway that you want to downregulate, which means decreasing the activity of the gene. Experiments in other species have shown to prolong lifespans up to 300 percent, so it should be no surprise that it's a common pathway found in centenarians who have a better insulin sensitivity. So by maintaining healthy sugar levels, you aren't activating this pathway, which can lead to longevity. As we'll discuss later with intermittent fasting, this system benefits from caloric restriction that can help extend the lifespan through a slower cell-growing metabolism.

- DAF-16 – This is part of the Fox0 family and is responsible for activating genes involved in controlling oxidative stress and longevity by integrating signals from different pathways to modulate the aging process.

- APOE – The protein encoded by this gene is a major apoprotein of the chylomicron, which means that it helps to transfer cholesterol to the appropriate systems, where it can be utilized in the production of male and female hormones, and cell membrane integrity. If there is a mutation present, there can be an increase in triglycerides and both plasma cholesterol and blood cholesterol, which is linked to cardiovascular disease and the hardening of arteries.

- hTERT – This gene helps aid in telomerase, which is responsible for maintaining the length of the telomeres in the cells. Studies in mice have shown that telomerase gene therapy can increase longevity without increasing the risk of cancer. The study also showed that expressing this gene had a positive effect on insulin sensitivity, osteoporosis, neuromuscular coordination, and other molecular biomarkers of aging.[201]

- mTOR – Just like p53, this too is a cancer pathway that influences longevity and aging. It's major role is as a nutrient sensor, like IGF-1. It has been implicated in many of the processes associated with aging, such as cellular senescence, immune response, cell stem regulation, autophagy (the function of the cell that removes unnecessary or dysfunctional components), mitochondrial function, and protein homeostasis.[202]

- kat7 – When experimenting on mice, a group of Chinese scientists inactivated the Kat7 gene and found that it extended the lifespan by about 25 percent. That doesn't mean that exact percent will translate to humans, but it's still impressive and another key insight to longevity. Kat-7 contributes to senescence in cells, so when the cells die, the tissue degrades, and aging occurs. By downregulating this gene, it can improve your lifespan and prevent aging.

- Ras – This is a pathway essential for regulating the health of the cell, as its expressed in all tissues. When a mutation occurs, it can activate a number of pathways associated with cell growth and ultimately lead to cancer. Ras is the most common oncogene in human cancer and found in around 20 to 25 percent of all human cancers.[203] It's also considered by many scientists to be the most dreaded oncogene, given its association with poor cancer prognosis and outcomes.

- Methylation also plays a role in longevity, as recent research has discovered a link between DNA, methylation, and aging.[204] Being over- or under-methylated can lead to premature aging or conditions that result in premature aging, so MTHFR, MTRR, MTR, BHMT, CBS, ACT, AHCY, and SUOX mutations can all contribute. These are all common mutations. You can refer to the chapter on methylation on how to prevent these genes from being expressed, and in the process, help combat premature aging.

CHRONOLOGICAL AGE VS. BIOLOGICAL AGE

"It is not how old you are, but how you are old."

That's a quote from French author Jules Renard, and I find it particularly relevant when speaking about the concept of biological age. We all know our chronological age, but that is just a number, and it's not a number that our bodies pay all that much attention to. Have you seen people who are a certain age but just look older? There have been articles comparing the mugshots of drug users over the years, and the way some of the people age in those photos is shocking.[205] A long-time methamphetamine or crack cocaine user in their thirties can easily look ten or twenty years older because of the wear and tear they put on their bodies. These various mugshots can show a significant deterioration over the years, and even though this is an extreme example, it shows how our environment and our behaviors can age our bodies so that our chronological age is not always the same as our biological age. Another factor to consider is your genomic age, which is purely your genes, and measured by methylation status. However, this too evolves into your biological age, since methylation can be influenced by diet, exercise, environment, and lifestyle choices. That goes to show how methylation can impact age. It really is connected to everything.

In my office, I have a medical device that accurately measures the biological age of my patients and has been used by prominent universities for research. BMI (body mass index) is another important factor linked to aging. Your BMI is based on height and weight. According to the National Institutes of Health, a BMI of 20 to 25 is preferred, 25 to 30 is overweight, 30 to 35 is obese, and over 35 is morbidly obese. It's important to note that BMI doesn't distinguish what type of weight, be it fat or muscle. To determine your actual body fat, you have to do a body fat scan. The higher your body fat content, the more susceptible you are to chronic conditions being expressed like cardiovascular disease, high blood pressure, high cholesterol, diabetes, colitis, inflammatory bowel disease, and Crohn's disease.[206] Diet, exercise, supplementation, and how you deal with stress can also impact your biological age. Sun exposure can lead to premature aging of the skin. I see this a lot in golfers. Sun, oxidation, and stress can all lead to skin wrinkling and the loss of its elasticity. All of this can impact the aging process.

I've studied the biological age of hundreds of patients, and there is definitely a pattern to the findings. It shouldn't be much of a surprise that the healthy patients who ate well, exercised regularly, and took care of their bodies, had a biological age younger than their chronological age. This was true of Alicia. When she was 74, her biological age was only 67 because she prioritized her health and took care of her body. The opposite was true as well, and the patients who smoked, consumed large quantities of alcohol, didn't exercise regularly, were under high amounts of stress, or lead an unhealthy lifestyle had a biological age up to seven years older than their chronological age. It's those unhealthy habits that can predispose your cells to premature aging. The good news is that unlike your chronological age, your biological age can change.

Elysium Health launched a Biological Age Test Kit that can be sent directly to your home, so you can provide a saliva sample and mail it back to the lab to be analyzed.[207] Thorne is another company that offers a similar test.[208] I'm sure more companies will follow suit, so this technology will soon be more readily available.

Technology continues to evolve at a rapid pace, and scientists are now learning about the ribosomal clock, which is a new way to measure your biological age. A ribosome is a collection of RNA molecules and proteins, and the main role of RNA is to convert the information stored in DNA to proteins. Right now, we're measuring biological age using the methylation portion of your genome, but this uses the ribosomal part of the genome. Ribosomal DNA, or rDNA, is the more conservative part of the genome, and it doesn't change often, so they believe it's a more accurate way to predict the age of the cell and measure your biological age. Scientists also hope that this will provide a better understanding of how environmental factors and lifestyle choices can influence aging.[209]

FUN FACT:

Women outlive men in 195 out of 198 countries, and on average by six years. However, in some countries that gap is as much as 11 years.[210]

THE POWERHOUSE OF THE CELL

The mitochondria is called the powerhouse of the cell because it produces energy in the form of ATP (adenosine triphosphate) from carbohydrates, fats, and proteins. Nearly every cell has thousands of mitochondria, and all of our cells, organs, and organ systems depend on ATP for energy. We need that energy throughout the day, and especially when exercising, because strenuous exercise can increase ATP demands 100-fold. Immune, cardiovascular, and neurological function all require energy, as does liver detoxification. Lack of sleep and stress can also deplete energy reserves, and a sedentary lifestyle, chronic conditions, and aging can limit your ATP production.

You want to preserve your body's energy supply, as there is a delicate balance between our body's energy demand and the supply provided by mitochondria. When the supply doesn't meet the demand, mitochondrial dysfunction can occur, which can lead to a variety of conditions and diseases that include Alzheimer's disease, Parkinson's disease, Huntington's disease, atherosclerosis, diabetes, metabolic syndrome, multiple sclerosis, lupus, type I diabetes, autism, schizophrenia, bipolar disorder, chronic fatigue syndrome, fibromyalgia, chronic infections, and cancer. [211]

There is a difference between mitochondrial dysfunction and mitochondrial disease, which is a chronic, genetic, and often inherited disorder where the body doesn't produce enough energy. It can be present at birth, or occur at any age, and it can impact almost any part of the body. Mitochondrial disease can result in low muscle tone, muscle weakness or pain, vision and hearing problems, learning disabilities, autism, heart disease, liver disease, kidney disease, gastrointestinal disorders, vomiting, cramps, diabetes, increased risk of infection, neurological problems, seizures, migraines, stroke, thyroid problems, respiratory problems, and dementia.[212]

An ACAT1 gene mutation, exercise, and diet can all directly impact mitochondrial function and the production of ATP. In addition to regular exercise, it's recommended that you eat small, frequent meals that contain meat, fish, nuts, fruits, and vegetables. But when diet alone cannot provide all of the proper nutrients, supplements such as CoQ10, Acetyl L—Carnitine, Alpha lipoic acid, and L-arginine can help to pick up the slack. Leucine, which is found in whey protein isolate, can help your body create more mitochondria, while creatine promotes ATP synthesis and muscle performance.[213] Mitochondria ATP from Pure Encapsulations is a great product that I recommend to my patients who need a proper energy boost.

FUN FACT:

Mitochondria have features that suggest they were formally independent organism, even with their own DNA. Those that carry out aerobic respiration have their own genomes.

THE CIRCULATORY SYSTEM AND YOUR LONG-TERM HEALTH

It starts with blood. The average adult has roughly 11 pints of it, which makes up about one-twelfth of our body weight. Blood is a collection of specialized cells that deliver oxygen, nutrients, and hormones while collecting waste, controlling temperature, and fighting infection to heal the body.

Blood is transported throughout the body through three main types of blood vessels: arteries, veins, and capillaries. Arteries carry oxygenated blood away from the heart, veins carry blood back toward the heart, while the capillaries are where gasses, nutrients, and waste between the blood and the tissues are exchanged. This circulatory system is how the heart maintains a steady supply of blood throughout the body. Any substance that is processed or used by our body, at one point or another, will be transported within the circulatory system, and it is a vast system. If you were to lay out all of the blood vessels in the body, they would stretch for over 60,000 miles, which is long enough to circle the earth two and a half times.[214]

The benefit of the foods we eat and the supplements we take are reliant on the circulatory system to deliver them where they need to go. As with everything, this also impacts our DNA. The cells have to be well-oxygenated and receive quality nutrition or they can malfunction or die prematurely. If you don't get the proper nutrients, your DNA sends the wrong signals, which leads to the production of the wrong proteins. When the template is faulty, so is the replication, so you have issues with future cell repair and division. This can lead to excessive organ damage that is much greater than the underlying stress. That makes the circulatory system directly linked to your genome.

One of the culprits affecting the integrity of the vascular system is inflammation and LDL cholesterol (or bad cholesterol), because it can harden and clog the arteries, which then restricts the blood flow. When you partially block the arteries, the heart needs to pump faster, which can lead to high blood pressure and enlarging of the heart. Given the percentage of block and location of the artery, the more work the heart has to do to meet the demands of the body and the lifestyle. Conditions like cardiovascular disease, arteriosclerosis (hardening of the arteries), and high blood pressure are conditions that can change the consistency of the arteries and the veins. This can also create issues that you might not think are connected to the circulatory system, like angina pectoris, varicose veins, sluggish lymphatic drainage, poor circulation, blood clotting, and thrombus formation. The body has a way of knowing which organs are more vital than others, so when blood flow is restricted by clogged arteries, organs and organ systems will suffer. That's why the goal is for the arteries to maintain their elasticity, and one of the best ways to do that is the natural way, through food and supplements.

Cardiovascular disease is the leading cause of death in Western countries, and responsible for 30 percent of deaths worldwide.[215] Research has shown the Mediterranean diet to be more beneficial for overall cardiovascular health compared to the traditional Western diet. The Mediterranean diet is also low-inflammatory, which is beneficial, since inflammation plays a role in coronary artery disease.[216]

Changing your diet, along with getting proper exercise and a healthy lifestyle, is optimal for improving cardiovascular health, but the following foods can help improve your body's circulation, so you can avoid common symptoms associated with poor circulation like pain and muscle cramps.

- Pomegranates
- Beets
- Radishes
- Berries
- Dark chocolate
- Fatty fish (Salmon)
- Citrus fruits
- Kale
- Brussels sprouts
- Coffee
- Chili peppers
- Cayenne pepper
- Cinnamon
- Turmeric[217]

What most of these foods have in common is that they are high in vitamins A, C, E, selenium, and zinc. Another food that has been shown to help combat coronary atherosclerosis (one of the most serious secondary manifestations of cardiovascular disease) is garlic, specifically aged garlic extract (and it's also available in supplement form), because it contains allicin, which reduces inflammation and has antioxidant benefits. Data also shows that garlic can help aid in reducing inflammation, so adding garlic to your diet or supplement regimen has significant benefits.[218] I take a garlic supplements myself, and often recommend it to my patients. Another great supplement that fights inflammation is Inflammacore from Orthomolecular Products.

As with everything in the body, our genes have an impact on the circulatory system. The one we know the most about is APOE and how it can predispose you to high cholesterol.[219] The CV Health Plus Genomics test from Genova Diagnostics looks at the APOE, MTHFR, Factor II, and Factor V genes. Scientists recently discovered the impact of a gene called SVEP1, which makes a protein that drives the development of plaque in the arteries.[220] If you have this gene, it means you are prone to the build-up of plaque, which can have a significant impact on your overall vascular health. PCSK9 is a cardioprotective, or heart protective, gene found in people with extremely low cholesterol, and that's a trait common to many centenarians.

Genomics is complicated, so none of this is cut and dry, and it doesn't all come down to one gene. Most cases of coronary artery disease are polygenetic, so there are 67 different gene variants that increase the risk of someone having coronary artery disease. Some of those genes are more common than others. I believe there are a lot of factors that go into aging, and still a lot we don't know about all of those genes, but APOE and SVEP1 are two that we do know more about.

You can take protective and preventive heart health measures by modifying your diet, supplementation, and lifestyle, but when you have your genome tested, you can find out if you have any of these genes that might predispose you to cardiovascular conditions. You can also undergo conventional blood tests and functional medicine tests. Genova Diagnostics' CV Health test is one I highly recommend because it provides a lot of information, while going above and beyond the conventional cholesterol test. Your functional medicine doctor has to order the test for you, but it's a good predictor of your overall cardiovascular health because there are factors other than cholesterol that need to be considered. One of the more publicized examples of this was former President Bill Clinton who had normal cholesterol levels and was given a clean bill of health only to end up having a quadruple bypass. Even his LDL bloodwork was within range. Apparently, it's the density (not only the size) of the LDL cholesterol particles that matters, and it's that kind of information a test like this, and functional medicine, can provide. I always tell my patients that LDL is like the bus that shuttles cholesterol to the arteries. LDL particles are the actual number of people on the bus, while LDL size is how big those people are. The more people, and the bigger they are, the higher the density, and the more damage they can cause to the arterial walls.

The CV Health test, which is a predictor of heart attack risk (along with diabetes and kidney disease), can show if there is any damage to the endothelial layer, which is the innermost of three layers of the blood vessels. The test measures the molecules to see the damage, and can then repair that layer with actual cholesterol, almost like you were putting plaster on a hole in the wall before you paint. This can prevent the arteries from leaking, but there are potential problems that can arise if you keep adding cholesterol.

THE HEALTHY CANNIBALIZATION OF OUR CELLS

Autophagy and apoptosis are both cell processes that are essential for maintaining homeostasis, or a state of stability and equilibrium that allows the body to function properly. On their most simple level, think of them like the body's way of taking out the trash and recycling. These are both very complicated and similar in a lot of ways, yet also quite different at times. We know how they work, and the research continues to evolve, but some of the mechanisms are still unclear. These are the basic definitions:

- Apoptosis: A Greek word meaning "falling away from," this dismantles damaged and unwanted cells from within to allow for programmed cell death and to remove faulty cells.
- Autophagy: A Greek word meaning "self-eating," this is part of our everyday cellular metabolism where healthy cells break down and

recycle damaged cells, and then salvage all of the nutrients and cell parts to be used elsewhere in the body to become new cellular components. It's a highly catabolic process (that promotes the breakdown of complex molecules) that also helps to restore the cellular energy balance when the cells are deprived of nutrients.

Apoptosis and autophagy are unlike the process of senescence, during which the cell remains metabolically active and alive. Both autophagy and apoptosis are involved in the housekeeping of the cell. They work together to do so and are stimulated by the same stressors, but they both slow down as we age, and can also decrease because of poor diet, which can cause toxins and cellular debris to build up and impair cellular function. Either too much or too little of either can result in various health issues, such as heart disease, autoimmune diseases, neurodegenerative diseases, metabolic disorders, liver disease, aging, and many types of cancer, which is why manipulation or autophagy plays a major role in being able to manage chronic disease.[221]

During this process of autophagy, some parts of the cell can be recycled, and the others are broken down and eaten up by the cell, so the cell essentially eats itself. The process is essential to cellular function by maintaining healthy cell components and balance, so they can retain their energy and function as intended. Since every cell in the body contains components that contribute to key metabolic function, this process is necessary to achieving optimal health.

There are over 36 genes related to autophagy and two major pathways or signal sensors. In general, autophagy can be classified as either mTOR dependent or independent. The mTOR pathway is considered a master regulator of cell health, insulin management, cell proliferation, protein synthesis, and nutrient metabolism. It's also a great nutrient sensor, and when inhibited in caloric restriction, it stimulates autophagy. Hypoxia, cellular stress, oxidative stress, ROS, and pathogen infections from viruses, parasites can all activate autophagy to break down those nutrients and use them to create more proteins or a new cell. Inhibition of mTOR has led to increased life expectancy, while drugs such as rapamycin is considered to be an mTOR inhibitor, while lithium and the amino acids glucosamine and mannosamine can induce independent mTOR autophagy.

You always want to consult a physician before taking any medication, but the following drugs have been found to induce autophagy:

- Metformin: This diabetes drug that can improve anxiety in some cases promotes autophagy.
- Sirolimus (or Rapamycin): This induces autophagy by inhibiting mTOR.
- Fentanyl: This synthetic opioid pain medication induces autophagy via activation of the ROS/MAPK pathway.
- Carbamazepine: This drug used to treat epilepsy and neuropathic pain induces autophagy.
- Imatinib: This chemotherapy medication induces autophagy in chronic leukemia cells.
- Bortezomib: This anticancer drug induces autophagy in head and neck carcinoma cells.[222]

Technically, autophagy is always occurring at a low level, but these conditions kick it into high gear. However, the more debris you have in your cell, the more difficult it is for apoptosis and autophagy to occur. Think about being stuck in an elevator for an extended period of time. It's much easier to breathe if you're in that elevator all alone compared to being stuck in that elevator with 20 people. You have to work harder to breathe. Autophagy works the same way, and if the cell is too crowded with debris, that can not only make the process inefficient, but it can also lead to mutations. This is yet another reason why the detox is so important because it can help rid the cells, tissues, organs, and organ systems of unnecessary toxins and debris, so the processes of autophagy can occur naturally and be effective.

If you suffer from chronic conditions, such as inflammation, you naturally want to increase autophagy to recycle and remove cellular debris to limit potential DNA damage. It can protect against certain psychiatric disorders, neurodegeneration, infectious diseases, inflammation (it can actually decrease or increase inflammation when needed), and it can increase muscle performance and increase energy balance in the cell.[223]

Increasing autophagy can also lead to longevity and help prevent chronic conditions, such as cancer. Studies have shown that mice genetically engineered to have impaired autophagy had increased rates of cancer. While you want to increase autophagy if you have a history of cancer in your family, and during the early stages of cancer, well-established cancer uses the process of autophagy to feed itself—the cancer actually breaks down the cell and feeds on the sugar. Whether you want to induce or inhibit autophagy all depends on what type of cancer you have, what stage it's in, and how it's being treated. However, here are some natural ways you can stimulate autophagy.

It's very difficult to measure autophagy unless you do a lab test, and even then, you often have to measure other factors that are directly connected to autophagy, such as inflammation, since they can lead to chronic conditions that decrease autophagy. Research continues to evolve, but there are many different compounds that have been shown to epigenetically increase autophagy, including genistein (found in soybeans), resveratrol (found in grapes, peanuts, and berries), EGCG (found in green tea), triptolide (found in thunder god vine), curcumin (found in turmeric), sulforaphane (found in cruciferous vegetables), pterostilbene (found in almonds, grapes, and blueberries), quercetin (found in red onion, honey, and tomato), methyl jasmonate (found in apples), gossypol (found in the cotton plant), polyphenon B (found in green tea), corynoxine, cedrol (found in the essential oil of conifers), amala extract (found in Indian gooseberry), black hoof mushroom, European black nightshade extract, East Indian sandalwood oil, neferine (from the Indian lotus), anacardic acids (found in the shell of cashew nuts), Astin B, and Oridonin (purified from the herb rabdosia rubescens).[224]

Additional ways to naturally trigger autophagy include:

- Diet and nutrition, specifically the ketogenic diet.
- Exercise, especially aerobic exercise where you create stress by physically exerting the body for an extended period of time.

- Supplements, particularly fish oil with Omega 6 and Omega 3 fatty acids. Vitamin D and NAD are also known to increase autophagy.
- Sleep. The circadian rhythm is also linked to autophagy.
- Coffee. Studies have shown that coffee increased autophagy in mice.[225]

Just as there are ways to increase autophagy, there are also numerous ways to decrease autophagy. Studies have shown the following substances have been found to decrease autophagy: Eugenol, Bafilomycin A1, Elaiophylin, Oblongifolin C, Matrine, along with the drugs Wortmannin, 3-methyladenine, Spautin-1, Clomipramine, Lucanthone, and Chloroquine.[226] Remember that this isn't necessarily a bad thing, nor does it mean you should avoid these substances. It's another reminder why it's so important to consult with your doctor before taking or discontinuing any medication or supplement.

It's important to note that both neurons (located in the brain and other parts of the nervous system) and cardiomyocytes (in the heart muscle) live for decades and don't undergo either autophagy or apoptosis as often, which is why it's important to keep them as healthy as possible. But it's not always healthy to increase autophagy. There are some neurodegenerative diseases that attack the nervous system, such as Parkinson's, where you actually want to inhibit autophagy because the diseases increase it more than necessary. Those conditions aside, at the end of the day, it all comes down to improving your cellular health and protecting your DNA, so you want to naturally trigger autophagy and apoptosis.

It's for these reasons that autophagy is another contributing factor to longevity, and recent animal studies have backed this up. When autophagy was activated in mice, their lifespan was extended an average of 17.2 percent, which is the equivalent of increasing the human lifespan from 78.5 to 92 years. [227] Researchers noticed an improvement in the animal's overall health as they aged as well, including lower body weight, increased insulin sensitivity, improved metabolic health, and resistance to oxidative stress, but when autophagy was inhibited, the animals no longer experienced the same longevity and health benefits.

There is no way to prevent our cells from aging, but through healthy diet, exercise, lifestyle, and frequent detox, we can stimulate autophagy that allows our bodies to naturally clear the waste and cellular debris to keep cells functioning properly and to increase longevity.

INTERMITTENT FASTING

Another way to trigger autophagy is through intermittent fasting, which has been shown to reverse aging and elongate the telomeres, which adds to longevity. It can also downregulate and reduce many of the anti-aging pathways listed above, including IGF-1. Studies in rats have shown that intermittent fasting increased their lifespan 36 to 83 percent longer.[228] In primates it has been shown to delay the onset of long-lasting age-related diseases like cardiovascular disease, type 2 diabetes, degenerative diseases, and cancer.[229] There are different methods of fasting, but here are some of the most popular:

- The 16/8 Method: This involves skipping breakfast and only eating during an 8-hour window, while fasting for the remaining 16 hours.
- Eat-Stop-Eat: This requires fasting for 24 hours one or two times per week.
- The 5:2 Diet: Here, on two nonconsecutive days per week you consume only 500 to 600 calories, and eat normally the other five days.[230]

Everyone is different, so you have to find the method that works best for you. Given the physical and mental demands everyday life can put on us, I'm more in favor of intermittent fasting, where you stop eating for 16 hours a day. If you're apprehensive, or the idea of not eating for a long period of time doesn't appeal to you, I tell my patients to pick one day a week to fast, preferably a weekday. Stop eating around 6 p.m., and then don't eat again until 10 a.m. the following morning. If you find that it's harder for you to refrain from eating at night and easier in the morning, you can adjust that scale accordingly. The point is to give your system a break. Try to make that last meal a plant-based meal and keep the portion small. Maybe eat some hummus, pita, beans, and a vegetarian taco. Keep it light. Prolonged fasting is more intense and harder for some people to stick to. For my patients who are curious, I recommend that they start by picking one day a month, preferably over a weekend, and giving it a shot.

No matter what method you choose, it will require a little bit of discipline at first, but you might be surprised how quickly your body gets used to it, and by design, you can't help but naturally eat less, which will help you lose weight and boost your metabolism. The only catch is that you can't overcompensate and overeat after the fast. You also want to refrain from drinking caloric-heavy liquids, so stick to water. Some experts recommend drinking coffee because it can help quell hunger. If you plan to skip breakfast, keep in mind that it's still best to take your supplements with food, so plan to do that later in the day with your first meal.

Fasting isn't only beneficial for aging and weight loss; it can help reduce health risks, such as multiple sclerosis, intestinal disorders, and some cancers. It can improve heart health, cognitive performance, and sleep problems; help regulate glucose; protect against Alzheimer's disease; and reduce the risk for cardiovascular disease.[231]

On the days you aren't fasting you can create an ultra-longevity booster to regulate your epigenome through diet. Foods such as broccoli, cabbage, garlic, cruciferous vegetables, green tea, cheese, butter, parsley, thyme, peppermint, basil herb, celery, artichoke, and curcumin from turmeric can stimulate longevity. Combine those foods with intermittent fasting and you get the best of both worlds.

REDUCING INFLAMMATION

When it comes to longevity and aging, inflammation plays an essential role because it's both the cause and symptom of so many diseases. Most all diseases have an inflammatory component, so being able to limit and control inflammation is the secret natural path to longevity.

Acute inflammation is the body's reaction to trauma, injury, infection, irritation, and a food or chemical allergy. This can lead to pain, swelling, and redness as blood vessels rush to the infected area. This is the body's natural healing response. Fever is another response to infection, as an increase in body temperature helps to fight bacteria. This leads to faster breathing, increased heart rate, and sweating to increase blood and oxygen flow, while removing toxins.[232]

When healing doesn't occur, this can lead to chronic inflammation, which is a much more significant long-term problem because chronic inflammation can damage the cell membrane, which means that it can affect the cell by making it susceptible to viruses, bacteria, and free radicals. Certain inflammatory diseases lead to the production of ROS and also RONS (reactive oxygen and nitrogen species) that can damage DNA, create cell division, cause mutations, and even damage some of the repair pathways, creating long-term damage.

Depending on the degree of inflammation, the cells might be beyond repair. These damaged cells can send signals to neighboring cells and tissues to create further inflammation. When the cell is compromised, so is our DNA, which is how chronic inflammation can lead to the deterioration of tissue, organs, organ systems, and eventually aging. This can become a vicious cycle that can lead to chronic disease. Common inflammatory conditions include:

- Osteoarthritis
- Rheumatoid arthritis
- Atherosclerosis
- Fibromyalgia
- Multiple sclerosis
- Psoriasis
- Bronchitis
- Asthma
- Type 2 diabetes
- Lupus
- Gout
- Hay fever

- Crohn's disease
- Cancer
- Heart disease
- Alzheimer's disease
- Ulcerative colitis[233]

Some of these conditions can ultimately lead to cancer if not properly treated:[234]

- Asbestosis and silicosis can lead to mesothelioma and lung carcinoma.
- Bronchitis can lead to lung carcinoma.
- Cystic bladder inflammation can lead to bladder carcinoma.
- Gingivitis can lead to oral squamous cell carcinoma.
- Inflammatory bowel disease, Crohn's disease, and ulcerative colitis can lead to colorectal carcinoma.
- Skin inflammation can lead to melanoma.
- Gastritis and ulcers can lead to gastric adenocarcinoma and MALT lymphoma.[235]

Inflammation is also one of the main precursors to weight gain, because it can cause:

- Insulin resistance.
- Oxidative stress.
- Appetite deregulation.
- Production of free radicals.
- Breaking down of joint tissue.

Weight gain also releases hormones that lead to more inflammation that creates a vicious cycle that some struggle to emerge from. In many cases, it's not weight gain that's the problem as much as it is the inflammation that needs to be addressed.

Whenever I talk about DNA damage, regardless of the cause, I always think about detox and antioxidants as a way to repair that damage, and you want to continue practicing healthy habits even after the detox is complete.

The best way to reduce susceptibility to inflammatory-related disease and weight gain is through proper diet and exercise. Intermittent fasting has also been shown to reduce inflammation. In addition to antioxidants, this is also where prebiotics, probiotics, and a healthy and robust autophagy system come into play. They can restore the health of your microbiome, and inflammation, oxidation, and the microbiome are all connected.

Certain drugs like ibuprofen can block some of the inflammation pathways, but not all of them, which is why ibuprofen is not effective all the time. The same is true about nutrition, which is why diet plays such a crucial role in combatting inflammation. You want to gravitate towards foods rich in vitamin A, vitamin C, vitamin E, bioflavonoids, bromelain, naringin, and also quercetin and methionine because they can slow down histamine release. Here's a basic breakdown of what to eat and what to avoid.

INFLAMMATORY FOODS TO AVOID:
- Citrus fruits
- Wheat
- Eggs
- Shellfish
- Dairy
- Chocolate
- Potatoes
- Tomatoes
- Peppers
- Eggplant
- Gooseberries
- Rhubarb
- Zucchini

ANTI-INFLAMMATORY FOODS TO EAT:
- Plums
- Peaches
- Pumpkins

- Squash
- Beetroot
- Strawberries
- Kiwi
- Sweet potatoes
- Squash
- Broccoli
- Kale
- Dark berries
- Avocados
- Sesame seeds
- Pumpkin seeds
- Sunflower seeds
- Onions
- Kelp
- Tuna
- Mackerel
- Herring
- Sardines
- Salmon
- Chicken
- Tofu
- Pineapples
- Nuts

When it comes to measuring acute inflammation, there are five physical signs:

1. Redness
2. Heat
3. Swelling
4. Pain
5. Loss of function

Even though there are some markers that can help identify inflammation, the symptoms are often nonspecific or not easy to identify, which can make it difficult to properly diagnose. However, your doctor can also conduct a physical exam and look at your bloodwork from the conventional lab tests to look for elevations in WBC, neutrophils, eosinophils, CRP, ESR, PCT, fasting insulin, HbA1c, serum vitamin D, serum ferritin, and red cell distribution width (RDW).

Cyrex Lab has an excellent new test called "Lymphocyte Map" which measures 29 inflammatory biomarkers, including cytokines, since inflammation increases the levels of cytokines. Another great test from Cyrex Lab is called "Multiple Autoimmune Reactivity Screen" measures predictive antibodies, some of which may appear up to ten years before the clinical onset of a disease. "GI Effects," a stool test by Genova Diagnostics, measures the levels of vitamin D, fatty acid profile, calprotectin, and lactoferrin, which can be a sign of inflammation. Genova Diagnostics also offers a serum and urine test called NutrEval which measures over 120 biomarkers and assesses the body's functional need for antioxidants, vitamins, minerals, essential fatty acids, amino acids, digestive support, and other specific nutrients.

SUPPLEMENTATING FOR LONGEVITY

NAD (nicotinamide adenine dinucleotide) is a coenzyme found in every living cell. It helps to convert what we eat into energy. The problem is that NAD declines roughly 50 percent between ages 40 and 60.[236] Stress, alcohol, lack of exercise, and poor sleep can also deplete NAD, so boosting levels can slow down the aging process and lower the risk of age-related conditions. There are NAD, NADH, and NAD+ supplements that have been shown to slow down and elongate the telomeres.[237] Here are two of the better ones:

- Elysium Basis
- Elevant Prime

These supplements tend to be on the expensive side. I don't recommend NAD supplements for anyone who is currently fighting cancer, has a history of cancer, or is genetically predisposed because they can be counterproductive. The reason is because cancer cells keep dividing uncontrollably and never enter the stage of senescence, or cell death. In other words, cancer cells keep dividing but the telomeres don't shorten, so you don't want to take supplements that elongate the telomeres because there is a fine line between anti-aging and cancer cells when it comes to telomeres.

Other common longevity supplements include:

- ASTAXANTHIN (Astaxanthin from Pure Encapsulations): This helps support the natural antioxidant defenses of the skin and joins while promoting healthy immune and cardiovascular systems. Astaxanthin is also found in Thorne Omega fish oils. This has also been found to switch on the FOXO3 gene in mice.[238]
- TELOS95: This is a brand-new supplement that helps to reduce inflammation and fight free radicals in the body.[239]
- TA-65z: A rare, plant-based supplement that can help to rebuild the telomeres and slow down cellular aging.
- RASPBERRY EXTRACT: Raspberries are loaded with phytochemicals and have a wide range of health benefits, specifically regulating the expression of anti-aging genes and downregulating the insulin IGF pathway, which is common in most centenarians.[240] (As part of "Indigo Greens" from Orthomolecular.)
- INDOLE 3 CARBINOL: I3C (Metagenics, Pure Encapsulations, and Thorne): Naturally found in vegetables, I3C has been shown to improve breast health, support prostate metabolism, detoxify the intestines and liver, and support the immune system, and studies have shown that it has extended the health of autoimmune mice.
- MODIFIED CITRUS PECTIN (MCP from Vital Nutrients or PectaSol from Econugenics): This is a complex polysaccharide that derives from the peel and pulp of citrus fruits. It helps to promote a healthy immune system by protecting healthy cells, tissues, and organs from the deterioration that naturally occurs during the aging process.

- RESVERATROL (Vital Nutrients): Found in red wine, grape skins, grape juice, and mulberries, Resveratrol is a polyphenolic compound that may act as an anti-aging agent to increase lifespan, in addition to promoting healthy organ function, supporting cardiovascular health, and maintaining normal cell growth.
- GREEN TEA EXTRACT (Vital Nutrients): This is rich in flavonoids and catechins that can enhance the immune system by promoting antioxidant activity. Green tea can support cardiovascular health, maintain cholesterol levels, and contribute to healthy cell function.
- GREEN TEA PHYTOSOME (Thorne): This is green tea with a phospholipid nutrient to enhance the bioavailability and absorption of the nutrients.
- CURCUMIN (Vital Nutrients): I really like their phyto-curcumin brand, which is curcumin with phosphatidylcholine, a phospholipid to enhance the bioavailability and absorption of curcumin.
- RESVERACEL (Thorne): This combines NAD and resveratrol with a phospholipid to enhance the bioavailability and absorption of the nutrients.

The good news is that some common and core supplements that you might already be taking also promote aging and longevity, such as:

- Multivitamins
- Vitamin A
- Vitamin C
- Vitamin E
- Vitamin D3
- Zinc
- DHEA
- CoQ10
- Fish oil
- Selenium
- Chromium picolinate

- Glutathione
- Melatonin

FUN FACT:

Researchers have discovered a significant connection between higher intelligence measured during childhood and youth with longer life and better long-term health.[241]

LONGEVITY HACKS

1. *The Power of Green Tea*

Green tea leaves (and also grape seeds) have catechins, which are a class of flavonoids (plant-based chemicals) that not only work as a powerful antioxidant, but help protect plants from environmental toxins, repair damage, and give foods like wine, tea, and chocolate their color and taste.[242] By drinking two cups of green tea a day, some experts believe you can help protect against cancer and cardiovascular disease. A 2018 study found that regular green tea-drinkers maintain lipoprotein (healthy) cholesterol later in life when most see a decrease. Green tea has also been shown to protect the body from free radicals, inhibit tumor growth, and benefit overall gut and brain health.[243]

2. *Don't Forget to Laugh*

The natural killer cells (NK cells) are a type of lymphocyte that boost your immune system by combating bad microbes, and have been shown to help fight the spread of cancer. It's been reported that these NK cells actually respond to your mood. When you're happy, they multiply, and one of the most significant emotions is laughter.[244] Act happy and find ways to laugh, and you might be adding years to your life.

3. *Make Meditation a Habit*

Meditation has also been linked to lowering cholesterol, blood pressure, and blood sugar, which can naturally lead to a longer lifespan. It can reduce stress and create a sense of calm and peace, which is a natural way to elevate your overall well-being.[245]

4. *Hyperbaric Oxygen Therapy*

I've said it throughout, but oxygen equals life, so any way you can help the oxidation of the cell will improve your genes and overall health. That's why hyperbaric oxygen therapy (HBOT) has become more common and is available at various spas and longevity clinics. The process involves getting pure oxygen into your body while sitting in a pressurized chamber for extended periods. Studies have shown that HBOT has extended the telomeres, improved the health of the tissues themselves, and can significantly impact the aging process. However, the participants in the study conducted five 90-minute sessions per week over three months, so it's also a significant commitment.[246]

FACT:
Better-educated and better-paid people live longer, on average, than those with less education and lower incomes in the United States. And this gap is widening according to a 2015 National Academies of Sciences, Engineering, and Medicine report. [247]

AGING REMAINS A COMPLEX PROCESS

There isn't just one thing you can do, or one gene connected to aging. I've seen patients with mutations that predispose them to certain cancers who also have the beneficial FOXO3 mutation. Nothing is black or white. There are so many factors involved. However, that's part of what I believe gives you an advantage because you have more ways to potentially influence your body and your genome, so you can approach it from different angles. If you have the FOXO3 gene, that's great, but if you don't, there is a chance you might have one of the other genes linked to aging. It's a multi-disciplinary approach, and on top of all that, there are still accidents and events completely out of our control that can occur.

We all have pluses and minuses as certain genes are turned on and off. That means that we have strengths and weaknesses, but when you have your genome analyzed, you become more aware of those pluses and minus, which means that you can take steps to improve those weaknesses. In other words, you have control over the way your genes behave. And there isn't just one gene or pathway responsible for longevity; it's cumulative.

THE FUTURE OF GENOMICS

IT HAS BEEN 30 YEARS SINCE THE HUMAN GENOME PROJECT WAS INITIATED. At the time, many predicted that the project would fail, but the opposite occurred. I've said it multiple times, but it's worth repeating that genomics is the gift that keeps on giving. And it's not just advancements in genomics that can revolutionize modern medicine and the way we look at health—it's all the different "omics." These include transcriptomics (study of the complete set of RNA transcripts), nutrigenomics (study of the relationship between diet and gene expression, or how your genotype affects your nutrient levels), proteomics (study of proteins), microbiomics (study of microbial cells), metabolomics (study of small molecules), and pharmacogenomics (study of the relationship between drugs and gene expression, or how your genotype affects your response to drugs).

When a patient of mine learned that his insurance would no longer cover his blood-thinner medication, he was forced to switch from a brand name to a generic version. It wasn't long before he experienced some very serious side effects. We ran his genome and learned that he had genes that predisposed him to side effects of that specific medication. If he knew beforehand, he could have avoided the issue. That's why out of all the benefits of genomics, I believe prevention is the most significant. Personalized medicine is taking on a whole new shape, and every year, scientists accumulate more data, which leads to more insight, and more opportunity for us to unlock the power of our genes.

Some wonder if that knowledge is too powerful and fear that genomics is becoming the science of playing God. That's the criticism being leveled at technology capable of designing human babies. The 1997 sci-fi film *Gattaca* depicted a world where children are conceived through genetic selection. Twenty-five years later, that world is very much within our grasp. Genome-editing tools can genetically alter a fetus in vitro for specifically selected traits that can influence eye color, gender, and disease risk. Obvious ethical hurdles aside, it wouldn't be surprising if some version of this happens in the near future. But where do we draw the line, and who draws it?

Scientists have already been able to use CRISPR technology to genetically engineer pigs whose tissues and organs have the qualities necessary for human transplantation. Given the overwhelming need for organs, these xenotransplants can save many, many lives. Some experts predict that safe and effective tissue and organ transplantation is only years away.[248]

Gattaca isn't the only movie that once seemed far-fetched that could become reality. *Jurassic Park* was a mega hit when the first installment was released in 1993. Over the next 25 years, it not only became a successful franchise, but science has advanced to the point where the technology at the root of the concept is within our grasp, albeit on a smaller scale. It's still not possible to bring dinosaurs back from extinction, since DNA can only survive for roughly a million years, and dinosaurs were long gone by then.[249] However, scientists in Siberia are working on the Pleistocene Park initiative to build a prehistoric zoo using ancient DNA to bring certain ecosystems and extinct species back to life. This is different than cloning, in that they use a similar species to bring an extinct species back to life. They would combine extinct mammoth DNA with current elephant DNA to create more of a hybrid animal. It can also be used to reintroduce the traits of some endangered species, such as the white rhino, back into the population.[250]

Science moves at such a rapid pace that we're learning what's possible before we can come to a consensus on the ethics, legalities, and privacy associated with this advanced technology. Improvements can still be made when it comes to the way scientists worldwide store and share their data, but this is such a new science, we're all forced to figure out how this works as we go. And even that is starting to change. As more people voice concerns about the security of their raw data, some companies are stepping up to fill that void, such as Vivos Vault, an advanced company that offers DNA storage and security options. They collect your specimen, protect it, and save it for any future catastrophes.[251] This technology is even crossing over into our social lives. Geneticist George Church (a Harvard professor who is one of the leading authorities in the field, and on the advisory board of Elysium) has created a dating app called Digid8, which allows you to date according to your genes. Users have the option to match with individuals who don't have certain inherited diseases. It's a fascinating concept, but as expected, has come under heavy criticism.

One reason why these services are becoming more popular is because the cost of acquiring your raw data is exponentially decreasing. The cost today is significantly less than it was even a few years ago. Ten years ago, it cost over $100,000 to have your whole genome sequenced. Today it costs close to $1,000 and some experts predict that it won't be long before it only costs $100.

What else will be possible in the future? Junk DNA might be a thing of the past, and we might know the function of every single gene in our bodies. When you visit the doctor's office, your genomic information might be as readily available as your blood type. What will be the status of CRISPR/Cas9? Is it possible that we could live in a world without any genetic disease? How long will the average human being live? Can what we learn about how our genes aid in therapies and treatments to the point where it increases our average life span?

The sky is the limit, but the main obstacle is lack of education, and it's a significant obstacle given how complex the subject matter. This technology is not easy for the average person to understand, but great efforts have been made by the educational community to begin teaching some of these concepts at the high school and college levels. Despite these efforts, this is all still very new, so even many medical doctors and educators don't understand the realities of genomic analysis. I know that I never would have become informed had I not gone back to school to earn my certification in genomics from Stanford University. It was a sacrifice, and required time away from my family, but that two-year commitment was well worth the investment for myself, my family, and my patients. As soon as I started to implement that information into my own practice, I saw results. That made me want to share those results, so others could benefit.

The goal is to bridge the gap, spread awareness, and make knowledge more accessible, so everyone can understand the potential of genomics and use these vast and powerful resources to improve their lives. But we still have a lot to learn, because in the last twenty years, scientists have discovered that the human genome is much more complex than anticipated. The single best way to continue learning about those complexities is by acquiring more raw data, specifically raw data from diverse demographics. We are a diverse species, but the majority of the raw data we have collected so far is from those of European descent. Getting more data from those of Asian and African descent can provide new insights. For example, certain African populations may be prone to sickle cell disease, but their genome protects against malaria. Once we can identify that gene, it can be used to protect others against malaria. Some populations in South Asia were found to have a very high pain threshold due to a variant in the SCN9A gene. Targeting that gene could lead to new treatment for severe pain.[252] That's why there are initiatives underway on different continents to raise awareness and acquire more raw data to help scientists come to better conclusions that will also make the technology more accessible and affordable. The pangenome is the collection of all the DNA sequences that occur in a species, and that is the big-picture goal.

Genomics is a fascinating field, and I continue to learn more every single day. It really is like opening up Pandora's Box. A week doesn't go buy where I don't read a new article about a topic or a possibility that further expands my mind. Even though the possibility of resurrecting the dead and designing babies is intriguing, that's not what interests me the most. It's the possibilities of prevention and what that means for the future of the human race that I find the most compelling.

With genomics, we all have a choice. We aren't helpless anymore. We have the ability to find out if we carry a gene that predisposes us to a certain condition, and we can do something about that. Genomics completes the picture. It allows us to trace particular problems back to the original instruction manual to see where those genetic instructions might be off. We can then fix the issue at the source. Imagine how empowering it is, when you're 20 or even 40 years old, to know that you can take measures to control your destiny in ways that weren't possible a generation earlier. Genomics can revolutionize how we approach personal health and the health care industry. If used responsibly, genomics will be a massive step forward for humanity.

APPENDIX

A<small>LL OF THE PRODUCTS</small> I <small>RECOMMEND IN THIS BOOK ARE AVAILABLE FOR</small> purchase on my site:

https://www.drmichaelswellness.com/store

There are also separate links for Metagenics and Full Script:

https://mmichael.metagenics.com

https://us.fullscript.com/welcome/mmichael

A HISTORY OF DNA AND GENETICS

When looking toward the future, it's impressive to learn how close we are to having the technology to design an entire human being trait-by-trait. The ethics might be questionable, but the science is nothing short of miraculous. It's equally impressive when looking back to see how we arrived at this point and the technological advances that were strung together by brilliant scientists, dating all the way back to the 1700s when a Swiss naturalist named Charles Bonnet first introduced the concept of genetic inheritance. He first suggested that there is a miniature human being within each sperm. During conception, this minuscule human being fuses with the female egg and develops into an infant.

THE FATHER OF GENETICS

Between 1856 and 1866, an Augustinian friar and scientist named Gregor Mendel discovered the concept of recessive and dominant alleles of DNA molecules by breeding pea plants. He kept a close eye on the shape of the pod, height of the plant, color, position of the flower, and the shape of the seed. Mendel then published a paper in 1866 in which he described the action of certain invisible factors that result in such visible and predictable changes. We now know that those invisible traits he was talking about were genes. Mendel has since become known as the father of genetics.

THE IDENTIFICATION OF NUCLEIN

In 1869, only a few years after the publication of Gregor Mendel's paper, a Swiss physiological chemist named Friedrich Meischer had made arrangements with a local infirmary to receive all of their puss-drenched bandages, so he could research the protein components of the white blood cells. That's when he discovered a mysterious substance that was high in phosphorous content and resistant to protein digestion. This was something new. He might not have realized it at the time, but the discovery would be a huge breakthrough, because what he came to know as nuclein was really deoxyribonucleic acid or DNA—but it would take the scientific community over 50 years to recognize the importance of his work.

THE EUGENICS MOVEMENT

Eugenics attempted to improve the genetic composition for all of humanity through selective breeding to promote positive traits throughout the generations. The idea was first promoted by Sir Francis Galton, a British scholar related to Charles Darwin, who believed an elite society was comprised of people with good genetic makeup. Opinions were divided, and his plan was never implemented due to ethical concerns. When the movement reached the United States in the nineteenth century, the goal was to identify negative traits in the current generation and prevent them from developing in the next generation. The movement gained momentum and led to the creation of the ERO (Eugenics Records Office) in 1911, destined to survey families and track down their histories. Strict immigration rules were put in place to sterilize individuals with poor traits, so they could not be passed down to the next generation. In the twentieth century, 33 states prepared sterilization plans to implement for the mentally ill and those suffering from alcoholism, criminality, blindness, deafness, and promiscuity. The movement slowly lost all of its credibility by World War II.

THE REDISCOVERY OF MENDEL'S THEORIES

In 1900, the community of scientists finally acknowledged the work of Gregor Mendel, sixteen years after he passed away, when Dutch geneticist and botanist Hugo de Vries, German geneticist Carl Erich Correns, and Austrian botanist Erich Tschermak Von Seysenegg all independently rediscovered Mendel's theory, providing more relevance to the previous experiments. Meanwhile, it was the work of biologist William Bateson in Great Britain who brought Mendel's work into the limelight, but since it often conflicted with that of Charles Darwin, it received opposition, thus preventing Mendel's theories from being incorporated into evolutionary theory for three more decades. Danish geneticist and botanist Wilhelm Johannsen would clarify that the distinction between a characteristic and its determinant was not consistent, as Mendel and his followers believed. He would also name the determinants "genes." Soon after, an American geneticist and zoologist named Thomas Hunt Morgan was the first to locate the genes on chromosomes and published a popular picture that looked like beads on a string.[253]

ASSOCIATION OF MENDEL'S THEORY WITH A HUMAN DISEASE

In 1902, an English physician named Sir Archibald Edward Garrod became the first man to associate Mendel's theory with human disease. He researched a human disorder called alkaptonuria. He collected family history along with urine samples from his parents to support his study. He concluded his investigation by claiming that alkaptonuria was a recessive disorder. Garrod published *The Incidence of Alkaptonuria: A Study in Chemical Individuality*, which turned out to be the first-ever account on recessive inheritance in human beings.[254] Still, scientists realized that more research was needed to uncover the link between DNA and genetic diseases.

DNA IDENTIFIED AS THE "TRANSFORMING PRINCIPLE"

By the 1940s, it was commonly understood that genes are enzymes that help in controlling metabolic functions. They were also considered simple protein particles. However, it wasn't until 1944 when a Canadian-American immunochemist named Oswald T. Avery identified nucleic acid present in all living organisms. This nucleic acid would later turn out to be the deoxyribonucleic acid or DNA. Avery would later join forces with two other brilliant scientists named Maclyn McCarty and Colin MacLeod to purify almost 20 gallons of bacteria. They soon realized that the substance they were searching for wasn't a carbohydrate or protein but was nucleic acid instead. After further analysis, they recognized it as DNA.[255]

FIRST PHOTOS OF CRYSTALIZED DNA FIBERS

Rosalind Franklin, an English chemist and X-ray crystallographer, working at King's College trying to improve X-ray crystallography, became the first person to photograph crystallized DNA fibers. She was able to determine the different dimensions of DNA strands and also the helix structure. J.D. Bernal described Franklin's photos as "the most beautiful X-ray photographs of any substance ever taken." The photographs taken by Franklin were later used by Raymond Gosling to produce the first crystals of DNA.

THE DOUBLE HELIX

In 1951, an American molecular biologist named James Watson visited Cambridge University in England, where he met Francis Crick, a British molecular biologist, and together they studied the DNA structure. They found that the DNA was arranged as a double-standard helix made up of A, T, G, and C, which were duplicates of one another and arranged in a head-to-tail configuration. They published their findings in the prestigious scientific journal *Nature* in 1953, and were later awarded a Nobel Prize for their efforts in physiology and medicine in 1962 along with Maurice Wilkins.

HUNTINGTON'S DISEASE

In 1983, scientists discovered a rare inherited and fatal condition where the nerve cells in the brain begin to break down. Symptoms include loss of muscle, spasms, poor coordination, amnesia, confusion, depression, hallucination, anxiety, and mood swings. Huntington's disease became the world's first-ever genetic disease. People typically start to see symptoms in their 30s and 40s, and there is no cure. Most patients survive 10 to 25 years after the onset of the illness.

BREAST CANCER & OVARIAN CANCER GENE DISCOVERED

In 1990, the King Laboratory at UC Berkeley provided the first known evidence of the BRCA1 gene that produces tumor-suppressing proteins. BRCA2 was discovered two years later. When these genes are mutated, there is a higher risk of developing breast cancer and ovarian cancer. Each of these mutations can be inherited from either parent, and there is a 50 percent chance that a child inherits this gene mutation from a parent who carries the mutation. Women with the altered gene have a 50 to 85 percent chance of developing breast cancer by the age of 70 and a 60 percent chance of developing ovarian cancer by the age of 85.[256]

DOLLY THE SHEEP

In 1996, after 277 attempts, British developmental biologist Ian Wilmut and his colleagues at the Roslin Institute in Scotland cloned Dolly the Sheep, the first mammal cloned by a process known as nuclear transfer. Dolly died in 2003 at the age of six from a lung affection that is not believed to be linked to the cloning process.

FIRST HUMAN CHROMOSOME DECODED

In 1999, after an international collaboration between scientists in the United States, England, Japan, France, Germany, and China, chromosome 22 became the longest, continuous stretch of DNA ever decoded. It was chosen because it was small in size and associated with several known diseases.

GENETIC CODE OF FRUIT FLY DECODED

Scientists had been studying fruit flies to better learn about traits and genes in the hope that it would further their understanding of the internal workings of humans. In 2000, they finally broke the genetic code of the fruit fly and were surprised to learn that 60 percent of the fly's genes matched up with human genes.

THE INTERNATIONAL MOUSE GENOME SEQUENCING CONSORTIUM

In 2002, the mouse was the first mammal to have its full genome sequence completed. The mouse genome may be 14 percent smaller than the human genome, but it's 95 percent similar to ours. Two years later, in 2004, the rat genome was published, which is still smaller than the human genome, but larger than the mouse genome.[257]

THE HUMAN GENOME PROJECT

In 1990, the U.S. Department of Energy and the National Institutes of Health (NIH) collaborated with countries all over the world, including England, China, and Germany to launch the Human Genome Project. It took 13 years, and cost $3 billion, but they accomplished the gargantuan task they set out to achieve when mapping all of the DNA in a human cell and identified roughly 20,000 to 25,000 genes. It's 99.9 percent accurate and was two years ahead of schedule. Craig Venter, PhD, the CEO of Celera Genomics, played a large role in speeding up the human genome project. That same year, the ENCODE project was launched by the National Human Genome Research Institute and set out to identify and characterize all of the genes in the human genome

THE 1,000 GENOMES PROJECT

First launched in 2008, the 1,000 Genomes Project was completed in 2018, and succeeded in sequencing 100,000 genomes from patients affected by rare disease and cancer. The following year, the first comprehensive analysis of cancer genomes was published, including lung cancer and malignant melanoma.[258]

GENOMICS AND THE LAW

After George H. Bush signed into law the Genetic Information Nondiscriminatory Act (GINA) in 2008 to forbid employers from discriminating on the basis of genetics, the U.S. Supreme Court ruled in 2013 that naturally occurring DNA cannot be patented.

COVID-19

Following the 2020 global pandemic, the genome of the SARS-CoV-2 virus was sequenced.

NOTES:

———

BIBLIOGRAPHY

INTRODUCTION

1   Wang Y, He J, Ma TJ, et al. *GSTT1* Null Genotype Significantly Increases the Susceptibility to Urinary System Cancer: Evidences from 63,876 Subjects. *J Cancer*. 2016;7(12):1680-1693. Published 2016 Jul 26. doi:10.7150/jca.15494. https://www.ncbi.nlm.nih.gov/pmc/articles/PMC5039389/#:~:text=The%20results%20suggested%20that%20the,CI%3D1.05%2D1.22

2   Servick, Kelly. "Embryo experiments take 'baby steps' toward growing human organs in livestock." Science. https://www.sciencemag.org/news/2019/06/embryo-experiments-take-baby-steps-toward-growing-human-organs-livestock

3   McFarling, Usha Lee. "Near the campus cow pasture, a scientist works to grown human organs – in pigs." STAT. https://www.statnews.com/2017/10/20/human-pig-chimera/

CHAPTER 1

4   Goldfeder RL, Wall DP, Khoury MJ, Ioannidis JPA, Ashley EA. Human Genome Sequencing at the Population Scale: A Primer on

High-Throughput DNA Sequencing and Analysis. Am J Epidemiol. 2017;186(8):1000-1009. doi:10.1093/aje/kww224. https://www.ncbi. nlm.nih.gov/pmc/articles/PMC6250075/#:~:text=From%20this%20 13%2Dyear%2C%20%243,found%20in%20humans%20(8).

5   Limer, Eric. "Researchers Cram 700 Terabytes of Data into One Gram of DNA.." Gizmodo. https://gizmodo.com/researchers-cram-700-terabytes-of-data-into-one-gram-of-5935929

6   "What is a gene?" From Genetics Home Reference., Medline Plus. https://medlineplus.gov/genetics/understanding/basics/gene/#:~:text=An%20international%20research%20effort%20called,one%20inherited%20from%20each%20parent.

7   Gibbons, Ann, "Bonobos Join Chimps as Closest Human Relatives" Science., June 13, 2012. https://www.sciencemag.org/news/2012/06/bonobos-join-chimps-closest-human-relatives#:~:text=Ever%20since%20researchers%20sequenced%20the,them%20our%20closest%20living%20relatives.

8   Annunziato, A. (2008) DNA Packaging: Nucleosomes and Chromatin. Nature Education 1(1):26. https://www.nature.com/scitable/topicpage/dna-packaging-nucleosomes-and-chromatin-310/

9   Starr, Dr. Barry. "A Long and Winding DNA." KQED, February 2, 2009. https://www.kqed.org/quest/1219/a-long-and-winding-dna#:~:text=Each%20human%20cell%20has%20around,miles%20away%20from%20the%20sun.

10   Ramsey, Lydia; Lee, Samantha. "Our DNA is 99.9% the same as the person next to us – and we're surprisingly similar to a lot of other living things." Business Insider Australia, May 7, 2016. https://www.businessinsider.com.au/comparing-genetic-similarity-between-humans-and-other-things-2016-5

11   Stanford Center for Professional Development. Stanford Genetics and Genomics Certificate. Slide 142.

12   "Genetics vs. Genomics Fact Sheet." National Human Genome Research Institute. https://www.genome.gov/about-genomics/fact-sheets/Genetics-vs-Genomics#:~:text=All%20human%20

beings%20are%2099.9,about%20the%20causes%20of%20diseases.

13   Blanco, Daniel Bastardo. "Our Cells Are Filled with 'Junk DNA' – Here's Why We Need It." Discover, August 13, 2019. https://www. discovermagazine.com/health/our-cells-are-filled-with-junk-dna-heres-why-we-need-it

14   Makalowski, Wojciech. "What is junk DNA, and what is it worth?" Scientific American, February 12, 2007. https://www. scientificamerican.com/article/what-is-junk-dna-and-what/

15   Stanford Center for Professional Development – Genetics and Genomics Certification Class, Genomics and other omics comprehensive essential. Complete presentation slides, page 239 of 321, "Big data storage challenges."

16   Genomics (2019). Fun Facts to Know. Retrieved from: https:// genomicstudy-dy.weebly.com/fun-facts.html

17   "Human Genome Project FAQ." National Human Genome Research Institute. https://www.genome.gov/human-genome-project/Completion-FAQ

18   Collins F. Has the revolution arrived?. Nature. 2010;464(7289):674-675. doi:10.1038/464674a https://www.ncbi.nlm.nih.gov/pmc/articles/PMC5101928/

19   Baidya, S. "25 Interesting DNA Facts." Facts Legend. 2014. https:// factslegend.org/25-interesting-dna-facts/

20   Stanford Genetics and Genomics Certificate – Stanford Center for Professional Development, Mutation: Small-Scale Changes, Course Slides.

21   C. Rachna. "Difference between Mutation and Variation." Bio Differences, December 21, 2018. https://biodifferences.com/difference-between-mutation-and-variation.html

22   "What Is Mutation?" Learn.Genetics. https://learn.genetics.utah.edu/content/basics/mutation/

23   Stanford University School of Engineering. "Nanobodies could help CRISPR turn genes on and off." Phys.org. February 25, 2021. https://phys.org/news/2021-02-nanobodies-crispr-genes.html

CHAPTER 2

24   Atkinson, Mark. "Mapping the 100 trillion cells that make up your body." The Conversation., September 26, 2018. https://theconversation.com/mapping-the-100-trillion-cells-that-make-up-your-body-103078

25   Fliesler, Nancy. "Presidential awardee explores epigenetics via slime molds, works, and more." Discoveries: Stories and news from Boston Children's, July 29, 2019. https://discoveries.childrenshospital.org/epigenetics-eric-greer-pecase/#:~:text=%E2%80%9CEpigenetics%20is%20what%20enables%20every,in%20response%20to%20their%20environment.

26   Lukaczer, Dan. Clinical Nutrition: A Functional Approach. IFM, January 2004.

27   Schriber, Michael. "The Chemistry of Life: The Human Body." Live Science, April 16, 2009. https://www.livescience.com/3505-chemistry-life-human-body.html

28   Yasko, Dr. Amy. Feel Good Nutrigenomics: Your Roadmap to Health. Neurological Research Institute, 1st edition. April 16, 2014.

29   Lam, Michael MD. "Methylation Disorder: What Is It and Why It Matters" Dr. Lam Coaching.

30   Dr. Amy Yasko. NRI: Neurological Research Institute

31   Samavat H, Kurzer MS. Estrogen metabolism and breast cancer. Cancer Lett. 2015;356(2 Pt A):231-243. doi:10.1016/j.canlet.2014.04.018. https://www.ncbi.nlm.nih.gov/pmc/articles/PMC4505810/

32   Nicolson GL. Mitochondrial Dysfunction and Chronic Disease: Treatment with Natural Supplements. Integr Med (Encinitas 2014;13(4):35-43. https://www.ncbi.nlm.nih.gov/pmc/articles/PMC4566449/

33   "What Exactly Is Methylation and Why Should I Care?" Nutrition & Your Genes. https://www.nutritionandyourgenes.com/what-is-methylation

34 Walsh, William J., PhD. "Methylation, Epigenetics, and Mental Health." https://www.walshinstitute.org/uploads/1/7/9/9/17997321/ methylation_epigenetics_and_mental_health_by_william_walsh_phd.pdf

35 Walsh, William J. PhD., "Methylation, Epigenetics, and Mental Health." https://www.walshinstitute.org/uploads/1/7/9/9/17997321/ methylation_epigenetics_and_mental_health_by_william_walsh_phd.pdf

36 Brookshire, Bethany. "Methylation turns a wannabe bumblebee into a queen." Science New., February 25, 2014. https://www.sciencenews.org/blog/scicurious/methylation-turns-wannabe-bumblebee-queen

37 Acharya, A. "DNA Day – Amazing things you did not know about your DNA." 2017. LinkedIn. https://www.linkedin.com/pulse/dna-day-amazing-things-you-did-know-your-anu-acharya

38 Adams, J. (2008) Obesity, epigenetics, and gene regulation. Nature Education 1(1):128. https://www.nature.com/scitable/topicpage/obesity-epigenetics-and-gene-regulation-927/

39 Skinner MK. A new kind of inheritance. Sci Am. 2014;311(2):44-51. doi:10.1038/scientificamerican0814-44, https://www.ncbi.nlm.nih.gov/pmc/articles/PMC4330966/

40 Nel-Thermaat, Ph.D., T.S (ABB), Russell, David, B.S., T.S. (ABB), "Epigenetics: You Are What Your Grandparents Age," Advanced Reproductive Medicine University of Colorado, October 12, 2016. https://arm.coloradowomenshealth.com/author/nelthemaatrussel

41 "Nutrition & the Epigenome." Learn.Genetics. https://learn.genetics.utah.edu/content/epigenetics/nutrition/

42 "Agouti Gene." ScienceDirect. https://www.sciencedirect.com/topics/neuroscience/agouti-gene

CHAPTER 3

43 "DNA Sequencing Costs: Data," *National Human Genome Research Institute.* Updated: December 7, 2020. https://www.genome.gov/about-genomics/fact-sheets/DNA-Sequencing-Costs-Data

44   "What are whole exome sequencing and whole genome sequencing?" From Genetics Home Reference. MedlinePlus. https://medlineplus.gov/genetics/understanding/testing/sequencing/#:~:text=These%20pieces%2C%20called%20exons%2C%20are,known%20as%20whole%20exome%20sequencing.

45   Regaldado, Antonio., "More than 26 million people have taken an at-home ancestry test." MIT Technology Review, February 11, 2009. https://www.technologyreview.com/2019/02/11/103446/more-than-26-million-people-have-taken-an-at-home-ancestry-test/

46   Powell, Kendall. "The broken promise that undermines human genome research." Nature, February 10, 2021. https://www.nature.com/articles/d41586-021-00331-5

CHAPTER 4

47   Lukaczer, Dan. Clinical Nutrition: A Functional Approach. Second Edition. The Institute of Functional Medicine. 2004.

48   Liska, DeAnn J. PhD., and Rountree, Robert, M.D. "The Role of Detoxification in the Prevention of Chronic Degenerative Diseases." Applied Nutritional Science Reports, Advanced Nutrition Publications, Inc. 2002.

49   "10 interesting facts about detoxing." Cabot Health, https://www.cabothealth.com.au/10-interesting-facts-detoxing/

50   Vikhanski, Luba. "Protecting the Brain from a Glutamate Storm." Cerebrum Dana Foundation, May 10, 2007. https://www.dana.org/article/protecting-the-brain-from-a-glutamate-storm/

51   Lukaczer, Dan. Clinical Nutrition: A Functional Approach. Second Edition. The Institute of Functional Medicine. 2004

52   "10 interesting facts about detoxing." Cabot Health, https://www.cabothealth.com.au/10-interesting-facts-detoxing/

53   Hanson, Carl. "12 Foods to Always Buy Organic (Plus 15 That Are Ok Conventionally Grown)." allrecipes, September 22, 2020. https://www.allrecipes.com/article/dirty-dozen-fruits-and-vegetables-to-buy-organic/

54   https://www.doctorsdata.com/comprehensive-drinking-water-analysis/

55   "Drug Development and Drug Interactions: Table of Substrates, Inhibitors and Inducers." FDA. https://www.fda.gov/drugs/drug-interactions-labeling/drug-development-and-drug-interactions-table-substrates-inhibitors-and-inducers

56   "10 interesting facts about detoxing." Cabot Health, https://www.cabothealth.com.au/10-interesting-facts-detoxing/

57   "10 interesting facts about detoxing." Cabot Health, https://www.cabothealth.com.au/10-interesting-facts-detoxing/

58   Graci, Sam. "21 Days to Crack the Code. Change your taste buds." Alive. April 24, 2015. https://www.alive.com/health/21-days-to-crack-the-code/#:~:text=All%20the%20bumps%20you%20see,narrower%20preference%20for%20food%20choices.

59   Jain, Naveen. "Microbiome: All Diseases Begin in the Gut. A Short Guide to Fixing Your Gut." Viome. 2017-2018.

60   Washington State University. "Connection Found Between Household Chemicals and Gut Microbiome," SciTechDaily, April 10, 2021. https://scitechdaily.com/connection-found-between-household-chemicals-and-gut-microbiome/

61   Frontiers, "New Species of Bacteria Discovered on Space Station May Possess 'Biotechnolgically Useful Genetic Determinants' for Growing Crops." SciTechDaily. March 18, 2021. https://scitechdaily.com/new-species-of-bacteria-discovered-on-space-station-may-possess-biotechnologically-useful-genetic-determinants-for-growing-crops/

62   Crew, Bec. "Here's How Many Cells in Your Body Aren't Actually Human." Science Alert, April 11, 2018. https://www.sciencealert.com/how-many-bacteria-cells-outnumber-human-cells-microbiome-science#:~:text=Luckey%2C%20who%20estimated%20that%20there,human%20intestinal%20fluid%20-or%20faeces.&text=%22More%20recent%20estimates%2C%20he%20noted,30%20trillion%20and%20400%20trillion.

63   Jain, Naveen. "Microbiome: All Diseases Begin in the Gut. A Short

Guide to Fixing Your Gut." Viome. 2017-2018.

64   Emerson, Mark D. "Listen to Your Gut: Healing from the Inside Out." DocEmerson Lifestyle Medicine Program.

65   Emerson, Mark D. "Listen to Your Gut: Healing from the Inside Out." DocEmerson Lifestyle Medicine Program.

66   Jain, Naveen. "Microbiome: All Diseases Begin in the Gut. A Short Guide to Fixing Your Gut." Viome. 2017-2018.

67   "Product of pomegranate juice extract promotes pathway to brain health." The University of Rhode Island, URI News External Relations and Communications, March 15, 2016. https://www.uri.edu/news/2016/03/product-of-pomegranate-juice-extract-promotes-pathway-to-brain-health/

68   "10 interesting facts about detoxing." Cabot Health, https://www.cabothealth.com.au/10-interesting-facts-detoxing/

69   Passwater, Richard A. All About Antioxidants. Avery, January 15, 1998.

70   Winderl, Amy Marturana, C.P.T.; Todd, Carolyn L. "What Are Antioxidants and What Do They Actually Do for Your Body?" Self, August 20, 2020. https://www.self.com/story/what-antioxidants-are-and-actually-do

71   Winderl, Amy Marturana, C.P.T.; Todd, Carolyn L. "What Are Antioxidants and What Do They Actually Do for Your Body?" Self, August 20, 2020. https://www.self.com/story/what-antioxidants-are-and-actually-do

CHAPTER 5

72   Suglia, Elena. "Vanishing Nutrients." *Scientific American,* December 10, 2018. https://blogs.scientificamerican.com/observations/vanishing-nutrients/

73   Wallinga D. Today's Food System: How Healthy Is It? J Hunger Environ Nutr. 2009;4(3-4):251-281. doi:10.1080/19320240903336977. https://www.ncbi.nlm.nih.gov/pmc/articles/PMC3489133/

74   Ducharme, Jamie., "Black Licorice Warning: Why FDA Says Don't Eat Too Much on Halloween." Health, February 25, 2021. https://www.health.com/condition/heart-disease/black-licorice-bad-for-you

75   Collins, Sonya. "Avoid Carcinogens, Not the Grill This Summer." Cure. June 16, 2014. Summer 2014, Volume 13, Issue 2. https://www.curetoday.com/view/avoid-carcinogens-not-the-grill-this-summer

76   Edgson, Vicki., Marber, Ian. The Food Doctor – Fully Revised and Updated: Healing Foods for Mind and Body. Collins & Brown. Revised, Updated Edition April 1, 2004.

77   Gunnars, Kris, BSc. "20 Nutrition Facts That Should Be Common Sense (But Aren't)." healthline, January 18, 2019. https://www.healthline.com/nutrition/20-nutrition-facts-that-should-be-common-sense

78   "The Epigenetic Influence of the Mediterranean Diet." Metagenics Institute. https://www.metagenicsinstitute.com/blogs/epigenetic-influence-mediterranean-diet/

79   "Dietitian Sheds Light on Nightshade Vegetables." Samaritan Health Services, January 11, 2021. https://www.samhealth.org/about-samaritan/news-search/2021/01/11/are-nightshade-vegetables-bad-for-you-to-eat

80   "Lectins." Harvard T.H. Chan School of Public Health. https://www.hsph.harvard.edu/nutritionsource/anti-nutrients/lectins/

81   Stanford University. Center for Professional Development. Genetics and Genomics Certificate. Course slide 132. 2017.

82   Simopoulos, Artemis P., M.D.; Robinson, Jo. The Omega Diet: The Lifesaving Nutritional Program Based on the Diet of the Island of Crete. Harper Paperbacks. March 1, 1999.

83   Edgson, Vicki; Marber, Ian. The Food Doctor – Fully Revised and Updated: Healing Foods for Mind and Body. Collins & Brown. Revised, Updated Edition April 1, 2004.

84   "14 Facts People Don't Know About Nutrition." Ideal Nutrition,

September 24, 2017. https://idealnutrition.com.au/14-facts-people-dont-know-about-nutrition/

85   Stephan C. Bizal, DC. "Creating Customized Patient Wellness Programs." 1/1/2008.

86   Gunnars, Kris. "The 8 Most Popular Ways to Do a Low-Carb Diet." healthline, March 7, 2019. https://www.healthline.com/nutrition/8-popular-ways-to-do-low-carb#TOC_TITLE_HDR_2

87   "How does genetic makeup influence dietary responses to carbohydrate intake?" GB Health Watch. https://www.gbhealthwatch.com/Nutrient-Carbohydrate-Genes.php

88   "The Relationship Between Weight Loss and Genetics." Psomagen, March 23, 2020. https://psomagen.com/the-relationship-between-weight-loss-and-genetics/#:~:text=Harvard%20Health%20has%20found%20that,as%20much%20as%2080%25%20responsible

89   Dansinger, Michael, MD. "Low-Fat Diets for Weight Loss." WebMD, February 7, 2021. https://www.webmd.com/women/reducing-dietary-fat#1

90   Hellman, Andrew. "DNA vs. Diet: APOA2 Gene Interacts with the Environment to Affect Weight." The Tech Interactive. https://genetics.thetech.org/original_news/news121

91   "LCT gene." MedlinePlus https://medlineplus.gov/genetics/gene/lct/

92   "IgG Food Antibodies." Genova Diagnostics. https://www.gdx.net/product/igg-food-antibodies-food-sensitivity-test-blood

93   "What is Celiac Disease?" Celiac Disease Foundation. https://celiac.org/about-celiac-disease/what-is-celiac-disease/

94   "Collaborative Report Suggests New Classification For Gluten-Related Disorders." Beyond Celiac, February 8, 2012. https://www.beyondceliac.org/research-news/collaborative-report-suggests-new-classification-for-gluten-related-disorders/

95   "The Growth of Gluten Sensitivity and the Genetics Behind It." OmeCare, November 22, 2019. https://omecare.co/resources/blog/the-growth-of-gluten-sensitivity-and-the-genetics-behind-it/

96   Anderson, Jane., "Do You Need Specific Genes to Have Gluten Sensitivity?" verwellhealth, December 1, 2019. https://www.verywellhealth.com/gluten-sensitivity-genes-562967

97   Li J, Maggadottir SM, Hakonarson H. Are genetic tests informative in predicting food allergy? Curr Opin Allergy Clin Immunol. 2016;16(3):257-264. doi:10.1097/ACI.0000000000000268. https://www.ncbi.nlm.nih.gov/pmc/articles/PMC5407010/

98   https://www.cyrexlabs.com/CyrexTestsArrays/tabid/136/Default.aspx

99   Gunnars, Kris, BSc. "20 Nutrition Facts That Should Be Common Sense (But Aren't)." healthline, January 18, 2019. https://www.healthline.com/nutrition/20-nutrition-facts-that-should-be-common-sense

100   https://www.diabetes.org/diabetes/complications

101   "LNP Delivers CRISPR Directly to Mouse Liver, Dramatically Cuts Cholesterol Levels for Months." Genetic Engineering & Biotechnology News, March 2, 2021. https://www.genengnews.com/news/lnp-delivers-crispr-directly-to-mouse-liver-dramatically-cuts-cholesterol-levels-for-months/#:~:text=Their%20studies%20in%20mice%20demonstrated,months%20following%20a%20single%20injection.

102   "Dietary Supplements Market Worth $272.4 Billion by 2028 / CAGR 8.6 %, Grand View Research, February 2021. https://www.grandviewresearch.com/press-release/global-dietary-supplements-market

103   National Research Council (US) Committee on Mapping and Sequencing the Human Genome. Mapping and Sequencing the Human Genome. Washington (DC): National Academies Press; 1988. 2, Introduction. Available from: https://www.ncbi.nlm.nih.gov/books/NBK218247/https://www.ncbi.nlm.nih.gov/books/NBK218247/#:~:text=The%20human%20genome%20is%20thus,nucleotide%20on%20the%20other%20strand.

104   "Got a Minute? Survey finds a nation in a hurry" NBC News., May 28, 2006. https://www.nbcnews.com/id/wbna13014283

105 Saleh, Naveedm, MD. "Don't drink coffee with these vitamins," MDLinx, August 14, 2020. https://www.mdlinx.com/article/don-t-drink-coffee-with-these-vitamins/2OI25UJKhJQllHAjBlNNQU

106 Radhakrishnan R, Wilkinson ST, D'Souza DC. Gone to Pot: A Review of the Association between Cannabis and Psychosis. Front Psychiatry. 2014;5:54. Published 2014 May 22. doi:10.3389/fpsyt.2014.00054. https://www.ncbi.nlm.nih.gov/pmc/articles/PMC4033190/

107 Ehlers CL, Gizer IR. Evidence for a genetic component for substance dependence in Native Americans. Am J Psychiatry. 2013;170(2):154-164. doi:10.1176/appi.ajp.2012.12010113. https://www.ncbi.nlm.nih.gov/pmc/articles/PMC3603686/

108 Gunnars, Kris, BSc, "20 Nutrition Facts That Should Be Common Sense (But Aren't)." healthline, January 18, 2019. https://www.healthline.com/nutrition/20-nutrition-facts-that-should-be-common-sense

CHAPTER 6

109 "Aging and the Microbiome: What Happens When You Get Older?" *Atlas Blog*, October 31, 2020. https://atlasbiomed.com/blog/ageing-and-the-gut-microbiome/

110 "10 Surprising Facts About Supplements." Superior Supplement Manufacturing, 2020. https://www.superiorsupplementmfg.com/10-surprising-facts-abou-suppelments/

111 "What You Need to Know about Dietary Supplements" FDA, November 29, 2017. https://www.fda.gov/food/buy-store-serve-safe-food/what-you-need-know-about-dietary-supplements#:~:text=The%20U.S.%20Food%20and%20Drug,them%20to%20friends%20or%20family.

112 https://regenr8.pro/

113 Steelsmith, Laurie, Dr. "Why Are Some Vitamins and Supplements More Expensive Than Others?" The Upside. https://www.vitacost.com/blog/are-expensive-vitamins-better/

114 Levin, Sasha. "What Are Binders and Fillers?" Purity Products,

May 27, 2020. https://www.purityproducts.com/blog/binders-and-fillers#:~:text=When%20manufacturing%20any%20vitamin%20or,carrier%20vehicle%20for%20active%20ingredients.

115 https://www.consumerlab.com/

116 "Dietary Supplements Market Size, Share & Trends Analysis Report By Ingredient (Vitamins, Proteins & Amino Acids), By Form, By Application, By End User, By Distribution Channel, and Segment Forecasts, 2021 – 2028." Grand View Research, February 2021. https://www.grandviewresearch.com/industry-analysis/dietary-supplements-market

117 https://www.elysiumhealth.com/en-us/science/scientific-advisory-board

118 https://www.vitalnutrients.net/quality

119 https://www.ayush.com/

120 https://www.jarrow.com/sciencepanel

121 Thorpe, JR., "21 Things No One Ever Told You about Daily Vitamins." Bustle, June 8, 2019. https://www.bustle.com/p/21-facts-about-daily-vitamins-no-ever-tells-you-17907413

122 "Vitamin B12: What to Know." Nourish by WebMD. https://www.webmd.com/diet/vitamin-b12-deficiency-symptoms-causes#1

123 "Vitamin B12 Fact Sheet." National Institutes of Health: Office of Dietary Supplements. https://ods.od.nih.gov/factsheets/VitaminB12-Consumer/

124 "Vitamin D." NHS. https://www.nhs.uk/conditions/vitamins-and-minerals/vitamin-d/

125 Thorpe, JR. "21 Things No One Ever Told You About Daily Vitamins." Bustle, June 8, 2019. https://www.bustle.com/p/21-facts-about-daily-vitamins-no-ever-tells-you-17907413

126 "Cholesterol and Triglycerides: Eating Fish and Fish Oil," C.S. Mott Children's Hospital Michigan Medicine. https://www.mottchildren.org/health-library/hw114960#:~:text=If%20you%20take%20a%20medicine,of%20a%20fish%20oil%20supplement.

127 "Supplement Fact, 170310." CRN. https://www.crnusa.org/ sfacts-170310

128 Whelan, Corey, and Olsen, Natalie, R.D. L.D. ACM EP-C. "Fructooligosaccharides." healthline, December 15, 2017. https:// www.healthline.com/health/fructooligosaccharides

129 Certification Board for Nutrition Specialists and Michael J. Glade, Ph.D., FACN, CNS. 2002.

130 https://www.gdx.net/product/gi-effects-comprehensive-stool-test

131 Nongyao Kasatpibal, JoAnne D. Whitney, Surasak Saokaew, Kirati Kengkla, Margaret M. Heitkemper, Anucha Apisarnthanarak. Effectiveness of Probiotic, Prebiotic, and Symbiotic Therapies in Reducing Postoperative Complications: A Systematic Review and Network Meta-analysis. Clinical Infectious Diseases, Volume 64, Issue suppl_2, 15 May 2017, Pages S153–S160. https://doi. org/10.1093/cid/cix114

132 Norris, Taylor., Olsen, Natalie., R.D., L.D., CSM EP-C. "What's the Difference Between Soluble and Insoluble Fiber?" healthline, March 1, 2018. https://www.healthline.com/health/soluble-vs-insoluble-fiber

133 Nebert DW, Wikvall K, Miller WL. Human cytochrome P450 in health and disease. Philos Trans R Soc Lond B Biol Sci. 2013;368(1612):20120431. Published 2013 Jan 6. doi:10.1098/ rstb.2012.0431. https://www.ncbi.nlm.nih.gov/pmc/articles/ PMC3538421/

134 "Primary Coenzyme Q10 deficiency." MedlinePlus. https:// medlineplus.gov/genetics/condition/primary-coenzyme-q10-deficiency/

135 Tardiolo G, Bramanti P, Mazzon E. Overview on the Effects of N-Acetylcysteine in Neurodegenerative Diseases. Molecules. 2018;23(12):3305. Published 2018 Dec 13. doi:10.3390/ molecules23123305. https://www.ncbi.nlm.nih.gov/pmc/ articles/PMC6320789/#:~:text=Among%20its%20various%20 properties%2C%20NAC,a%20scavenger%20of%20oxidant%20 species.

136 Lukaczer, Dan. Clinical Nutrition: A Functional Approach. Second edition. The Institute of Functional Medicine, 2004.

137 "Vitamin E." National Institutes of Health Office of Dietary Supplements. https://ods.od.nih.gov/factsheets/VitaminE-HealthProfessional/#:~:text=Vitamin%20E%20is%20a%20fat,diseases%20associated%20with%20free%20radicals.

138 Thorpe, JR. "21 Things No One Ever Told You About Daily Vitamins." Bustle, June 8, 2019. https://www.bustle.com/p/21-facts-about-daily-vitamins-no-ever-tells-you-17907413

139 "Theanine." WebMD. https://www.webmd.com/vitamins/ai/ingredientmono-1053/theanine

140 "SAMe." Mayo Clinic. https://www.mayoclinic.org/drugs-supplements-same/art-20364924#:~:text=Generally%20safe,SAMe%20and%20prescription%20antidepressants%20together.

141 "Molybdenum." National Institutes of Health, Office of Dietary Supplements. https://ods.od.nih.gov/factsheets/Molybdenum-HealthProfessional/#:~:text=The%20top%20sources%20of%20molybdenum,teens%20and%20children%20%205B19%5D.

142 "Liquids Vs. Pills." Medicare Europe. https://medicare-europe.co.uk/science-clinical-data/liquids-vs-pills.html/#:~:text=Generally%2C%20supplements%20in%20liquid%20form,than%20most%20capsules%20and%20pills.

143 "Economic Impact Fact: More than 383k jobs." CRN Supplement Facts, September 30, 2016. https://www.crnusa.org/CRN-Supplement-Facts/September-30-2016

144 Thorpe, JR. "21 Things No One Ever Told You About Daily Vitamins." Bustle, June 8, 2019. https://www.bustle.com/p/21-facts-about-daily-vitamins-no-ever-tells-you-17907413

145 https://www.gdx.net/product/nutreval-fmv-nutritional-test-blood-urine#:~:text=The%20NutrEval%20FMV%C2%AE%20is,support%2C%20and%20other%20select%20nutrients.

CHAPTER 7

146 "Walking: Your steps to health." Harvard Health Publishing: Harvard Medical School, April 19, 2021. https://www.health.harvard.edu/staying-healthy/walking-your-steps-to-health

147 Haff, Gregory G., Triplett, Travis N. Essentials of Strength Training and Conditioning. Human Kinetics, Fourth Edition, November 16, 2015.

148 Collins, Ryan., Legg Timothy J., Ph.D., CRNP. "Exercise, Depression, and the Brain. healthline, July 25, 2017. https://www.healthline.com/health/depression/exercise

149 Markell, Jenny. "Can Listening to Music Improve Your Workout?" Health Research. https://www.center4research.org/can-listening-music-improve-workout/#:~:text=A%202010%20study%20led%20by,%2C%20productivity%2C%20or%20strength.%E2%80%9D

150 Quinn, Elizabeth, Pereira, Erin, PT, DPT. "Fast and Slow Twitch Muscle Fiber with Performance." verywellfit. June 10, 2020. https://www.verywellfit.com/fast-and-slow-twitch-muscle-fibers-3120094

151 Haff, Gregory G., Triplett, Travis N. Essentials of Strength Training and Conditioning. Human Kinetics, Fourth Edition, November 16, 2015.

152 Magee, Elaine, MPH, RD. "8 Ways to Burn Calories and Fight Fat." Nourish by WebMD. https://www.webmd.com/diet/obesity/features/8-ways-to-burn-calories-and-fight-fat#1

153 King's College London. "Scientists find link between genes and ability to exercise." ScienceDaily, 26 February 2020. <www.sciencedaily.com/releases/2020/02/200226171112.htm>.

154 "Physical exercise is not only important for your body's health – it also helps your brain stay sharp." brainHQ. https://www.brainhq.com/brain-resources/everyday-brain-fitness/physical-exercise/#:~:text=Exercise%20stimulates%20the%20brain%20plasticity,to%20grow%20new%20neuronal%20connections.

155 "The Odds of Injury: Genetic Testing and Sports." YouTube, uploaded by the Aspen Institute, June 28, 2019. https://www.

youtube.com/watch?v=0lC43vJqYic

156 "DNA Testing Could Be the New Moneyball For Sports." Mr. Feelgood. https://mrfeelgood.com/articles/dna-testing-could-be-the-new-moneyball-for-sports

157 "Exercise and immunity." MelinePlus, https://medlineplus.gov/ency/article/007165.htm#:~:text=Physical%20activity%20may%20help%20flush,system%20cells%20that%20fight%20disease.

158 Boham, Elizabeth. MD, MS, RD; and Hyman, Mark, MD. "Low T? 5 Steps to Boost Testosterone Naturally." The Ultrawellness Center. https://www.ultrawellnesscenter.com/2015/05/29/5-steps-to-boost-testosterone-naturally/

159 "Aromatase Inhibitors." The Institute for Functional Medicine. https://www.ifm.org/wp-content/uploads/Aromatase-Inhibitors-1.pdf

160 Boham, Elizabeth MD, MS, RD; and Hyman, Mark, MD. "Low T? 5 Steps to Boost Testosterone Naturally." The Ultrawellness Center. https://www.ultrawellnesscenter.com/2015/05/29/5-steps-to-boost-testosterone-naturally/

161 "Aromatase Inhibitors." The Institute for Functional Medicine. https://www.ifm.org/wp-content/uploads/Aromatase-Inhibitors-1.pdf

CHAPTER 8

162 "PCSK9 inhibition: A game changer in cholesterol management." *Mayo Clinic*. November 20, 2015. https://www.mayoclinic.org/medical-professionals/cardiovascular-diseases/news/pcsk9-inhibition-a-game-changer-in-cholesterol-management/mac-20430713

163 Kehr, Dr. Bruce. "Surf's Up: Use Your Genetic Code to Ride the Stress Wave with Ease. The COMT Gene." Dr. Bruce Kehr. DNA: I Am Who I Am… or Am I? https://drbrucekehr.com/comt-gene-test-stress-genetic-testing/

164 "25-hydroxy vitamin D test." MedlinePlus. https://medlineplus.gov/ency/article/003569.htm#:~:text=The%20normal%20range%20

of%20vitamin,30%20and%2050%20ng%2FmL.

165   "Vitamin D Deficiency." Cleveland Clinic. https://
       my.clevelandclinic.org/health/articles/15050-vitamin-d--vitamin-d-
       deficiency

166   "Vitamin D Deficiency." Cleveland Clinic. https://
       my.clevelandclinic.org/health/articles/15050-vitamin-d--vitamin-d-
       deficiency

167   Hancocks, Nikki. "Study: Elderly patients previously on
       vitamin D3 supplements more likely to survive COVID-19."
       NUTRAingredients.com. https://www.nutraingredients.com/
       Article/2020/11/04/Study-Elderly-patients-previously-on-vitamin-
       D3-supplements-more-likely-to-survive-COVID-19

168   Arnarson, Atli., BSc, PhD. "The Fat-Soluble Vitamins: A, D, E,
       and K." healthline., February 16, 2017. https://www.healthline.
       com/nutrition/fat-soluble-vitamins#:~:text=Fat%2Dsoluble%20
       vitamins%20are%20most,Vitamin%20D

169   Minadeo-Fox, Claudia. DDS. "Interesting Facts about Vitamin D."
       Health Inspired Dentistry, Whole Body Health & Wellness, August
       12, 2015. https://healthinspireddentistry.com/blogs/interesting-
       facts-about-vitamin-d/#:~:text=It%20is%20the%20only%20
       vitamin,getting%20enough%20from%20the%20sun.

170   Gardner, Dr. Aaron, BSc, MRes, PhD. "The Warrior Gene: 5
       Common Myths Debunked." MyGeneFood, November 12, 2020.
       https://www.mygenefood.com/blog/warrior-gene-5-common-
       myths/

171   Gardner, Aaron, Dr., BSc, MRes, PhD. "MAOA." GeneFood.
       https://www.mygenefood.com/genes/brain-and-mental-health-
       genes/maoa/

172   "Folic acid in diet." MedlinePlus, https://medlineplus.gov/
       ency/article/002408.htm#:~:text=Folate%20is%20a%20B%20
       vitamin,and%20added%20to%20fortified%20foods.

173   Meyers, Amy, M.D. "MTHFR Mutation: What It Is and What to
       Do About It." Amy Meyers M.D. https://www.amymyersmd.com/
       article/mthfr-mutation/

174 "MTR gene." MedlinePlus. https://medlineplus.gov/genetics/gene/mtr/

175 O'Connor, John. "Why Sulfur and the CBS Genes Are on My Nutrition Radar." MyGeneFood, November 17, 2020. https://www.mygenefood.com/blog/sulfur-cbs-genes-nutrition-radar/

176 Genovations. DetoxiGenoimc Profile. Genomic Assessments. Genova Diagnostics.

177 "Association of GSTM1 and GSTT1 Gene Deletions with Risk of Head and Neck Cancer in Pakistan: A Case-Control Study." Asian Pacific Journal of Cancer Prevention, 11(4):881-5, January 2010.

CHAPTER 9
178 https://www.bluezones.com/dan-buettner/

179 Calver, Tom and Stylianou, Nassos. "Nine facts about how long we live." BBC News, May 14, 2018. https://www.bbc.com/news/health-43726436#:~:text=1.,deaths%20in%20low%2Dincome%20countries.

180 O'Connor, C. (2008). Telomeres of human chromosomes. Nature Education 1(1):166. https://www.nature.com/scitable/topicpage/telomeres-of-human-chromosomes-21041/

181 Beyer AM, Norwood Toro LE. Telomerase: Location, Location, Location? Arterioscler Thromb Vasc Biol. 2018 Jun;38(6):1247-1249. doi: 10.1161/ATVBAHA.118.311054. PMID: 29793988; PMCID: PMC6028234. https://pubmed.ncbi.nlm.nih.gov/29793988/

182 Sahin E, Depinho RA. Linking functional decline of telomeres, mitochondria and stem cells during ageing. Nature, 2010, Mar 25;464(7288):520-8. doi: 10.1038/nature08982. PMID: 20336134; PMCID: PMC3733214.

183 "What is a telomere?" Your Genome, July 21, 2021. https://www.yourgenome.org/facts/what-is-a-telomere

184 Beyer AM, Norwood Toro LE. Telomerase: Location, Location, Location? Arterioscler Thromb Vasc Biol. 2018 Jun;38(6):1247-1249. doi: 10.1161/ATVBAHA.118.311054. PMID: 29793988;

PMCID: PMC6028234. https://pubmed.ncbi.nlm.nih.
gov/29793988/

185 "Telomere Analysis Technology. Results Report. Life Length, S.L.
www.lifelength.com, January 17, 2018.

186 Bernardes de Jesus B, Vera E, Schneeberger K, et al. Telomerase
gene therapy in adult and old mice delays aging and increases
longevity without increasing cancer. EMBO Mol Med.
2012;4(8):691-704. doi:10.1002/emmm.201200245. https://www.
ncbi.nlm.nih.gov/pmc/articles/PMC3494070/

187 Victor W.T. Liu, Paul L. Huang, Cardiovascular roles of nitric
oxide: A review of insights from nitric oxide synthase gene
disrupted mice. Cardiovascular Research, Volume 77, Issue
1, 1 January 2008, Pages 19–29. https://doi.org/10.1016/j.
cardiores.2007.06.024

188 Dambeck, Susanne. "Ten Astonishing Facts about Longevity."
Lindau Nobel Laureate Meetings, October 11, 2016. https://www.
lindau-nobel.org/ten-astonishing-facts-about-longevity/

189 Herskind AM, McGue M, Holm NV, Sorensen TIA, Harvlad B,
Vaupel JW. The heritability of human longevity: a population-based
study of 2,872 Danish twin pairs born 1870-1900. Hum Genet.
1996;96: 319-323.

190 University of Rochester. "Longevity gene' responsible for
more efficient DNA repair." Science Daily, 23 April 2019. www.
sciencedaily.com/releases/2019/04/190423133511.htm

191 "SIRT6 Overexpression Extends Lifespan in Mice." Genetic
Engineering & Biotechnology News, June 2, 2021. https://www.
genengnews.com/news/sirt6-overexpression-extends-lifespan-in-
mice/

192 Molina-Serrano D, Kyriakou D, Kirmizis A. Histone Modifications
as an Intersection Between Diet and Longevity. Front Genet.
2019;10:192. Published 2019 Mar 12. doi:10.3389/fgene.2019.00192.
https://www.ncbi.nlm.nih.gov/pmc/articles/PMC6422915/

193 Hasty P, Campisi J, Sharp ZD. Do p53 stress responses impact
organismal aging?. Transl Cancer Res. 2016;5(6):685-691.

doi:10.21037/tcr.2016.12.02. https://www.ncbi.nlm.nih.gov/pmc/articles/PMC6461382/

194   Baar MP, Brandt RMC, Putavet DA, Klein JDD, Derks KWJ, Bourgeois BRM, Stryeck S, Rijksen Y, van Willigenburg H, Feijtel DA, van der Pluijm I, Essers J, van Cappellen WA, van IJcken WF, Houtsmuller AB, Pothof J, de Bruin RWF, Madl T, Hoeijmakers JHJ, Campisi J, de Keizer PLJ. Targeted Apoptosis of Senescent Cells Restores Tissue Homeostasis in Response to Chemotoxicity and Aging. Cell. 2017 Mar 23;169(1):132-147.e16. doi: 10.1016/j.cell.2017.02.031. PMID: 28340339; PMCID: PMC5556182. https://pubmed.ncbi.nlm.nih.gov/28340339/

195   Stanford University. Understanding Cancer at the Genetic Level. Course lectures. https://online.stanford.edu/courses/xgen202-understanding-cancer-genetic-level

196   Stracquadanio, G., Wang, X., Wallace, M. et al. The importance of p53 pathway genetics in inherited and somatic cancer genomes. Nat Rev Cancer 16, 251–265 (2016). https://doi.org/10.1038/nrc.2016.15.

197   Slattery ML, Curtin K, Ma K, Edwards S, Schaffer D, Anderson K, Samowitz W. Diet activity, and lifestyle associations with p53 mutations in colon tumors. Cancer Epidemiol Biomarkers Prev. 2002 Jun;11(6):541-8. PMID: 12050095. https://pubmed.ncbi.nlm.nih.gov/12050095/

198   Yasuko Kitagishi, Mayumi Kobayashi, Satoru Matsuda, "Protection against Cancer with Medicinal Herbs via Activation of Tumor Suppressor." Journal of Oncology, vol. 2012, Article ID 236530, 7 pages, 2012. https://doi.org/10.1155/2012/236530.

199   Nebert DW, Wikvall K, Miller WL. Human cytochromes P450 in health and disease. Philos Trans R Soc Lond B Biol Sci. 2013;368(1612):20120431. Published 2013 Jan 6. doi:10.1098/rstb.2012.0431. https://www.ncbi.nlm.nih.gov/pmc/articles/PMC3538421/

200   Vitale G, Pellegrino G, Vollery M, Hofland LJ. Role of IGF-1 System in the Modulation of Longevity: Controversies and New

Insights From a Centenarians' Perspective. Front Endocrinol (Lausanne). 2019;10:27. Published 2019 Feb 1. doi:10.3389/ fendo.2019.00027. https://www.ncbi.nlm.nih.gov/pmc/articles/ PMC6367275/

201   Bernardes de Jesus B, Vera E, Schneeberger K, Tejera AM, Ayuso E, Bosch F, Blasco MA. Telomerase gene therapy in adult and old mice delays aging and increases longevity without increasing cancer. EMBO Mol Med. 2012 Aug;4(8):691-704. doi: 10.1002/ emmm.201200245. Epub 2012 May 15. PMID: 22585399; PMCID: PMC3494070. https://pubmed.ncbi.nlm.nih.gov/22585399/

202   Papadopoli D, Boulay K, Kazak L, et al. mTOR as a central regulator of lifespan and aging. F1000Res. 2019;8:F1000 Faculty Rev-998. Published 2019 Jul 2. doi:10.12688/ f1000research.17196.1. https://www.ncbi.nlm.nih.gov/pmc/ articles/PMC6611156/#:~:text=The%20central%20role%20for%20 the,as%20major%20determinants%20of%20longevity.

203   "Ras Pathway." addgene https://www.addgene.org/cancer/ras-pathway/

204   Johnson AA, Akman K, Calimport SR, Wuttke D, Stolzing A, de Magalhães JP. The role of DNA methylation in aging, rejuvenation, and age-related disease. Rejuvenation Res. 2012;15(5):483-494. doi:10.1089/rej.2012.1324. https://www.ncbi.nlm.nih.gov/pmc/ articles/PMC3482848/

205   https://abcnews.go.com/Health/photos/drugs-mugs-12999387/ image-12999422

206   Harper JW, Zisman TL. Interaction of obesity and inflammatory bowel disease. World J Gastroenterol. 2016;22(35):7868-7881. doi:10.3748/wjg.v22.i35.7868

207   https://www.elysiumhealth.com/en-us/index

208   https://www.thorne.com/products/dp/biological-age

209   Wang M, Lemos B. Ribosomal DNA harbors an evolutionarily conserved clock of biological aging. Genome Res. 2019;29(3):325-333. doi:10.1101/gr.241745.118. https://www.ncbi.nlm.nih.gov/ pmc/articles/PMC6396418/